THE BODY-MIND-SPIRIT LINKS TO HEALTHY AGING

THE BODY-MIND-SPIRIT LINKS TO HEALTHY AGING

Lillian L. Beeson
and
Mary Jane Dugan

Studies in Health and Human Services
Volume 46

The Edwin Mellen Press
Lewiston•Queenston•Lampeter

Library of Congress Cataloging-in-Publication Data

Beeson, Lillian L.
  The body-mind-spirit links to healthy aging / Lillian L. Beeson and Mary Jane Dugan.
      p. cm. -- (Studies in health and human services ; v. 46)
    Includes bibliographical references and indexes.
    ISBN-0-7734-7152-9
    I. Title. II. Series. III. Studies in health and human services (Lewiston, N.Y.) v. 46.

This is volume 46 in the continuing series
Studies in Health and Human Services
Volume 46 ISBN 0-7734-7152-9
SHHS Series ISBN 0-88946-126-0

A CIP catalog record for this book is available from the British Library.

The Edwin Mellen Press
Box 450
Lewiston, New York
USA 14092-0450

The Edwin Mellen Press
Box 67
Queenston, Ontario
CANADA L0S 1L0

The Edwin Mellen Press, Ltd.
Lampeter, Ceredigion, Wales
UNITED KINGDOM SA48 8LT

Printed in the United States of America

I dedicate this book to the memory of my parents, Ida Lois (Ball) and John R. Poe who struggled through the Great Depression but never lost sight of their goals to give their life and mine meaning. They taught me to choose hope over despair and to begin any revolution with self appraisal. I celebrate their courage and strength with everything that I accomplish. (Lillian L. Beeson)

This book is dedicated to Grandma Kaufman who raised me, nurtured me, and taught me how growing old can be fun; you just need a sense of humor. Also to Grandpa Kaufman who gave me unconditional love, husband Jerry whose support gives me strength, and to son Raymond who makes my life complete. (Mary Jane Dugan)

Table of Contents

Foreword

In the last one hundred years, average life expectancy in the United States has nearly doubled. At the same time, the proportion of the U.S. population over 65 grows ever larger as baby boomers continue to age. How ironic, given these circumstances, that our culture continues to worship and glorify youth to the detriment of our elderly.

Images of young people dominate our national psyche. Youthful images saturate every facet of the media. Beauty, fitness, power, wealth and intellect are among the positive attributes typically ascribed only to the young. On the other hand, media images of our aging population are relatively few and typically negative, emphasizing the loss of beauty, wealth, mental capabilities, and the like.

What a shame that we as a culture, and seniors in particular, continue to ascribe to the aging myth. We assume that, as we age, our bodies and minds will inevitably cease to function normally, and that we will ultimately become a burden to our families and society. Yet there is clear evidence that such decay is not inevitable at any particular age. Consider the fact that when 65 was established as the magical age for social security, it was because people who lived to such a ripe old age were not fully functioning and were truly incapable of caring for themselves. Today, most people in their sixties are fully functioning. Many continue to lead productive, fulfilling lives well into their seventies, eighties, even their nineties.

Too often, our fear of aging leads us to look for a quick fix for aging. Surgery to eliminate lines and wrinkles, or otherwise alter our appearance, and pills to alter our mental functioning are two of the obvious "fixes." More often than not, such quick fixes are ineffective or temporary and we again search for a painless way to stop the aging process. Instead of offering a quick fix, the

i

Wellness Model proposed by Drs. Beeson and Dugan represents a naturalistic, holistic, and common sense approach to aging.

This is an approach that is sound, both physically and psychologically. First, rather than beginning with the assumption that we should all strive to remain some perfect youthful age, the authors celebrate advancing age for what it represents. Here we have another unique phase in a life well lived, underscored by a vast store of knowledge acquired through a lifetime of experience. This is the time to enjoy the fruits of years of labor, focus on enjoying (rather than rearing) family, learn things that there simply was not time for in the busyness of youth, and share experiences with the younger generations.

In addition to celebrating the uniqueness of later life, Drs. Beeson and Dugan emphasize the connection between mind and body. Descriptions of psychological disorders typically include physical symptoms as well as disturbances of affect (mood), cognition (thought). Similarly, many physical disorders are accompanied by psychological symptoms. Thus, interconnectedness of mind and body is of paramount importance.

The Wellness Model is based on the fundamental necessity of maintaining both an active mind and an active body to facilitate health and well being. We have long known that an active body tends to be a healthy body. Increasingly we are finding that the same dictum holds true for our minds. Keeping the mind active has important benefits in staving off psychological disorders, mental deficiencies, and pathologies. People who stay active, both mentally and physically are less prone to some psychological disorders, like depression.

The Wellness Model is an important contribution in that it makes specific recommendations for maintaining a healthy active mind and body through the senior years. Typically, recommendations that are vague and nondirective are difficult to follow due to a high degree of ambiguity. When the doctor tells you to "stay off your feet," what does she really mean? The model described here does not suffer from such vagaries. Instead, each step of the model is discussed in detail, with many clear examples to guide the user.

The authors further acknowledge the necessity of tailoring the model to the needs of the individual. Certainly, different people have different preferences, in foods, in hobbies, and in physical activities. Further, physical disabilities or other existing medical conditions, in addition to age, may present some very real limitations to physical activities. Drs. Beeson and Dugan emphasize that an active lifestyle is not a one-size-fits-all proposition. Which activities are appealing and how much activity makes for an active lifestyle varies from one person to the next, and the authors make recommendations that can be tailored to fit any interest or level of ability.

This book has important implications for readers of all ages and abilities. Seniors who are currently inactive may take heart. There is ample research cited to demonstrate the benefits of adhering to the Wellness Model, even if you come to it later in life. Seniors who are already maintaining an active lifestyle may enjoy learning about the benefits they have already reaped! They may also add to their repertoire of physical activities from the many described in the text. Adult children with aging parents may use this as a tool either to get their parents moving or to keep them motivated to maintain both healthy minds and bodies. For younger adults, the Wellness Model provides a useful blueprint for healthy aging.

Ultimately, the choices we make about how we handle the aging process affect our quality of life. Drs. Beeson and Dugan point out the many directions these choices may take us, from physical activity to medications. They assert that the choices we make for the care and functioning of our bodies should be made carefully and not simply left in the hands of others. In the final analysis, we are each the guardian of our own wellness. Following the Wellness Model is a step in the right direction.

Debra K. Evans-Rhodes, Ph.D.
Penn State University

Preface

It is a fact that Americans are living longer and remaining active longer than ever before. There were over 50,000 Americans who had reached the age of 100 according to the <u>Statistical Abstracts</u> from the 1990 U. S. census data. The 2000 census will probably indicate an even greater number of centenarians but were not available at the time of this writing. The Baby Boomers are moving into their 50s and 60s and their numbers will change the political landscape on issues affecting the elderly. They have enjoyed health benefits which were not available to their parents such as polio vaccines, antibiotics, and freedom to pursue leisure activities away from the drudgery of factories or farms. Their longevity will place new strains on Social Security, health care services, and retirement arrangements since no former generations have lived so long. The U. S. Congress tried unsuccessfully during the Clinton administration to construct a national health policy that would serve both the old and the young without trading off the welfare on one group for the other.

We know that the central value in life does not derive from the number of years one survives, but rather the quality of life in relation to health, meaningful relationships and the power to maintain one's dignity. Further, we know that age alone is not the determining factor in people's perception of their satisfaction with life. Some individuals assess their quality of life by doing an inventory of socioeconomic status, health, and friends while others transcend the particulars of their life and embrace all of it with a philosophic grace regardless of wealth, health, or social networks. So satisfaction with life among the elderly is as individualized as it is among younger generations.

The authors of this book perceive that stereotypes and biases which portray the elderly as depressed, senile, or sick need to be redefined. The central idea of the work is that aging is a normal process and not a disease which needs to be treated by drugs or shunned by society as a plague to be avoided. A few individuals in our culture treat the elderly as untouchables, but the deficit is in their close-minded nature and certainly not the elderly who have survived to old age status.

The elderly members of America who are now in their 90s have watched their society change from the horse and buggy era to the jet age. Their generation survived the Great Depression, ushered in the Nuclear Age, and developed both radio and television–forces now considered more powerful as a social influence on moral development than education, religion, and parents in America. How can such a generation be considered dull? Their sacrifices and unwavering patriotism led us through the Great Wars–both World War I and II, and they have watched America march into the technocratic era of microchips and satellite space stations. We could learn a great deal from their tenacity and adaptability. Unlike the youth of the 90s called the X Generation, the elderly who are in their frail years now never seemed to lose sight of America's goodness and strengths.

The authors of this book have developed a Wellness Model which explains a healthy lifestyle that combines the mind, body, and spiritual unity which engenders generativity and renewal. This holistic approach is essential to individuals for a meaningful life that cultivates health, psychological well-being, and a link to other human beings and the universe. The model prescribes exercise, nutrition, life-long learning, and an active role in society throughout the lifespan. The deleterious effects of inactivity, dependence on drugs, abuse of alcohol and social isolation are addressed.

Since drug use and abuse is a major issue among the elderly, four chapters are devoted to discussing physical changes in the way the body absorbs, eliminates, and reacts to prescription and over-the-counter drugs as we age. The focus is on preventative measures like strength training, daily exercise, and alternative measures to maintain wellness. We believe that a life filled with friends and laughter are the best therapies to pursue daily. Genetic predispositions to disease or physical infirmities are not ignored in the chapters since heart disease, arthritis, diabetes, and other chronic disorders are commonplace among the elderly. While the prescribed model will not eliminate all of these factors, the measures recommended will delay or diminish the effects of such diseases.

Stress reduction and safety issues are discussed as measures to prevent accidents or hospitalizations. Even when individuals know the risk involved in certain actions such as walking on a wet floor or driving a car while the operator has multiple impairments, they will still engage in the behaviors. These issues are worthy of attention since medical costs are accelerating at an alarming rate and the elderly receive the greatest allocation of health dollars in the country.

The psychological barriers that separate the generations are illustrated throughout the book. Difficulties that result from the inability of professionals to communmicate with their clients, the reluctance of the young to communicate with their elders, and the intransigence of some elderly people toward all others are examined as root problems. Mass media contributes to the prevailing images of America's elderly. Portraits of ineffectual, impotent or confused persons in commercials, in literary characterizations, and in everyday jargon relegate our elderly to fringe social positions. Our book reexamines these attitudes and invites all readers to do the same. The real damage results from the internalization of these negative messages by the elderly who begin to accept the sick role assigned to them as they look to doctors and drugs to fix everything about their lives. Sometimes the problems are related to bereavement, loss of income, displacement from their homes, and fear of dependency upon others who may not be able to sustain them in their last years of life.

We urge that all individuals assume stewardship for the course of their life.

This means choosing healthy alternatives over dependence on drugs, inactivity, and disengagement from the mainstream of society. One does not have to be Mother Theresa, Grandma Moses, Pablo Picasso, or Senator Strom Thurman to bear witness to the talents that elderly people afford us. Yet the things that each of these well known individuals share is the drive to contribute to society in some way–charitable acts, art, and social change. The productive years are not confined to the first four or five decades of our lives. If we assume responsibility for our intellectual growth and health status, we can redefine the message of what old age really means in our culture. Many problems that were associated with aging are not inevitable results of chronological progression, but rather the effects of stress, smoking, misuse of drugs, poor diet, alcohol, lack of exercise, and unhappiness in interpersonal relationships. The Wellness Model explores these complex interrelationships along with the normal physical changes that accompany the aging process.

The book was truly a collaborative effort between the two authors, both of whom have taught in Gerontology programs; so, they researched the relevant areas, discussed the model, and wrote their chapters. Dr. Beeson wrote chapters one, five, seven, eight, nine, eleven, and fourteen. Dr. Dugan wrote chapters two, three, four, six, ten, twelve, and thirteen. Their combined experience in both the medical and educational fields have compelled them to try to put all of it together in an accessible manner for various readers. The holistic approach to aging encompasses both the strengths and weakness of people in advanced years but urges all readers to look at the whole person in their multi-dimensional personae. We cannot treat diseases until we understand the person standing before us and that entails more than a checklist of symptoms. The body, mind, and spirit are inseparable parts of the whole and anything that affects one affects the other in powerful ways.

Chapter 1

Introduction

Symbols that a society uses to represent ideas are derived from values, attitudes and beliefs about that particular concept. These symbols may possess inherently positive, negative or neutral images that can influence or direct certain responses. In America the images that symbolize aging are quite negative and the stereotypes of elderly people are tied to conventional wisdom, which portrays them as impoverished, senile, lonely, and powerless. This negativity culminates from various sources but the primary difficulty arises from the identification of elderly people as sick or in a terminal state and therefore patients who must be cured of some disease. The basic premise of this book is to establish that aging is a natural process and not an illness. What must change essentially is the national attitude toward elderly people so that we focus upon their functional strengths rather than their dysfunctions and stress wellness rather than illness.

Why do we view the developmental stages from infancy to early adulthood as exciting growth and the years from 35 on as years of decline? Even the best selling books have addressed middle age as beginning at 40, a time when we begin an inevitable decline or downward slide into illness or helplessness. The protagonists in these novels generally struggled with life's complexities until mid-life and then they accept notions of decline and loss. Dreams and high adventure are no longer portrayed for the middle aged characters; instead, their life is depicted as one of increasing anonymity and impotency. Frequently these middle aged characters are portrayed as confused, ineffectual, and out of the mainstream of life.

The *1996 World Almanac* recorded 3,080,165 people who were 85 years or older. [1] The *1995 Statistical Abstract* from the U.S. Department of Census recorded 50,000 people who were 100 years old--9,000 males and 41,000 females. [2] These figures ought to motivate us to find better visions for those great numbers between the dynamic under-forty generation and those who have demonstrated the coping skills to not only survive into old age, but to possess the grace and wisdom that comes from productivity and good living.

If you look at the symbols for the passage of time, you will find the new year arriving as a cherubic baby and Father Time leaving bowed and beaten. Frequently the old year looks like the grim reaper-death itself. The negative connotation that the life spectrum takes on in this culture is an example of propaganda that needs to be exposed for it is based upon false assumptions. The stereotypical view currently presents the early years as dynamic and magical and any stages after 40 as the slippery slope into death's door. Babies come into the world pure and curious processing stimuli from the moment of birth. Young childhood is touted as a time of rapid learning and self awareness. Adolescence is an awkward time between the shelter of childhood and the full flowering of identity in autonomous individuality. Early adulthood is characterized by choosing a mate, beginning a career, and creating a family unit. Negatively, as 35 to 45 approaches, black humor frequently paints a scenario of decline in creativity, productivity, sexuality and optimism. By 65, the age arbitrarily chosen as the year one becomes elderly, many individuals have bought into the social definitions or stereotypes of elderly people and they begin to play the sick role assigned to them. They become participants in the assumptions that they are "over-the-hill," supposed to be depressed, and ultimately withdraw from an active role in life. The negative self image inherent in this social role assignment means that some are less willing to use their talents; remain physically, mentally, and psychologically challenged; and engage in the social networks that gave them pleasure as young people.

The objective of this book is to offer a wellness model that prescribes an active participation by elderly individuals in the definition of their personhood and life rather than a willing embrace of patient status and death. Those who choose to follow the sick model will find themselves managed by others, inundated with drugs and invasive procedures, and ultimately dependent upon forces outside themselves for day-to-day living. We do not deny the finite nature of the human body; however, we do prescribe an infinite number of ways to preserve one's self identity and autonomy. Each individual must accept responsibility for his or her well being without delegating their welfare to doctors, family, quick-fix solutions or super-heroic measures.

We want to redefine AGE as America's Generation with Experience. We propose a wellness model of living which recognizes human potential at any age. The policy demands prevention, maintenance, and recovery. While we recognize the limitations that come naturally as we move from the crest of physical power into frailty, we urge everyone to resist the cultural imperative to be willing victims to social stereotypes at any age. Each individual can maintain physical strength and wellness by daily exercise, stress management, proper nutrition, and accepting the responsibility for one's own well being. Drugs are essential in some instances but there are no panaceas. In fact, drugs are frequently a double-edged sword. We have illustrated throughout the book how drugs are abused or misused by the elderly instead of giving the intended therapeutic effect.

A holistic approach to aging engages the unity of the mind, body, and spirit as we address the total person. The wellness model that we recommend combines these intellectual, physical, emotional, and spiritual components. A new body of research called psychoneuroimmunology (PNI) clearly indicates the impact that our mind has upon the body and includes the spiritual dimensions of happiness, optimism and friends as significant predictors of overall health. Clear links have been established between bad stress, those conditions or events that have negative consequences for us like loss of our job or a divorce, and suppression of the immune system. Researchers recognize good stress as those happy occasions that require us to adapt such as a wedding, a new baby, or a promotion and job transfer. These findings support the holistic approach to life that recognizes the interplay of influence between our thoughts, the response from our body, and long range effects on our health and happiness. The chapters and issues included in the book are outlined below.

(W) Walking and Waltzing

(E) Exercise alternatives

(L) Learn alternatives to drug therapy

(L) Listen to other options

(N) Necessary drugs only

(E) Eating proper foods–Nutrition an alternative to drugs

(S) Safety and precautionary measures

(S) Stress reduction techniques

(M) Management and control of drugs

(O) Overcome fears through education

(D) Drug and drug reactions education

(E) Enjoy have fun and play

(L) Laughter as internal jogging

The various aspects of healthful living will be discussed with these principles in mind:

1. **GENETICS**: Each individual manages their life given the genetic gifts and liabilities they have inherited. All things are not equal and some carry greater payoffs or risks.

2. **HAPPINESS**: Good fortune and living well are superior to any other therapies available. Drugs control not only diseased conditions, but individuals themselves. Ultimately the cure is often worse than the disease.

3. **RESPONSIBILITY**: Each individual is the architect of their day-to-day existence. Wise choices now are investments in future pay-offs in health, independence, and clarity of thought.

4. **KNOWLEDGE:** An enlightened individual is empowered to choose their own destiny. Education and knowing the risks or benefits of drugs, surgeries, and habits of living are essential for enlightened decision making at any age.

5. **INDEPENDENCE**: Through habits of living individuals create choices or alternatives that broaden their horizons throughout the life span. The more choices they have created, the better the investments in health, happiness, and quality of life overall.

We will discuss the natural changes in bodily functions which dictate special care. Body strength can be maintained into old age, and recovered to some extent through exercise. Pharmacology is not the answer to all problems that confront elderly people. In recent years an increased awareness of the negative effects of drugs on the elderly has contributed to regulations on all levels to seek more holistic practices toward recovery or control following illness. The individual must assume the primary responsibility for their lifestyle. Collaboration with family, physicians, and the community at large is essential.

6

Endnotes

1. <u>World Almanac and Book of Facts 1996</u>. (1995). Mahwah, N J: Funk and
    Wagnalls Corporation.

2. U.S. Department of Census. (1995). <u>Statistical Abstract of the United States</u>
    (115ed., p. 16). Washington, D.C.

Chapter 2

Walking & Waltzing

Have you ever driven down a highway and passed a convoy of vintage cars moving toward their designated shows? As they trudge down the road, they proudly display their shiny newly painted coats that radiate vibrant hues of fluorescent golds, siren reds, and glossy ebonies. One is struck with a sense of admiration and astonishment for their regal beauty and operable conditions. This antiquated fleet moves slower than most vehicles, but there is an ambience of pride, dignity, and nobility that emanates from their mere presence.

Although vintage vehicles are mechanistic wonders, they also can be compared with the human as a machine. One principal reason for the cars' mobility is the obvious fact that they have been kept in motion. It is unimportant that they do not move quickly, nor are their engines in vogue. The dominant component is these automobiles continue to use the mechanisms that remain, and do so with a kind of mortal dignity and pride. Similar to these vehicles, the human machine must "use it or lose it" meaning we must use our mobility or risk becoming inert or stationary, unable to move. [1] Our model for wellness recommends a renovation in attitude, expectations, and spirit toward the aging process, and endorses the proposition that being old does not portend a motionless and lifeless existence. Maggie Kuhn, the under 5 Foot tall 80 lb. founder of the Gray Panthers, was told by a friend that she was more spirit than body. [2] It is this spirit in aging Americans that needs to be refurbished. The human spirit is the gasoline or energy that provides the individuals with the will and vitality to survive. An uplifted spirit opposes the aging person's tendency to accept decline as a matter of course over which they have no control. Some degeneration is inevitable, but one need not become passive and helpless in life because others view them as old. The first step then is to "keep stepping" regardless of any alterations in agility, mobility, or speed.

Wellness is a lifestyle,[3] a concept that includes values and a positive approach to life. Spiritually, it is an attitude or belief that can propel the individual into a healthier mode. From a holistic perspective, the human body is one interacting unit consisting of three components; that of body mind, and spirit.[4] Thus, when the body is diseased or in a process of decline, a disharmony occurs that can trigger emotional and spiritual spin-offs. Therefore, if the spirit is low, there can be physical ramifications. On the other hand, humans also can possess a predisposition for healing or alleviating the symptoms of many conditions. Specific physical activities often serve as preventive measures that ward off many degenerative processes. Walking is one of those activities. It can energize the spirit, warm up the body's rigid muscles and joints, and activate the mind.

The difficult part lies with generating enough motivation to move or to do physical activities. Our model suggests that when physical activity is initiated a circular interactive motion energizes and unites the body, mind, and spirit. The spark plug or catalyst for initiating motion is the human spirit. This is the psychological or emotional impetus that generates the motivation or desire to be active. This driving force is the incentive that propels the individual into such activities as walking, waltzing, or even jogging. Therefore, a positive spirit is a necessary ingredient for combating the kind of aging declines that may make movement painful. At times it is easier and maybe less painful to remain immobile. The propelling factor that overcomes a stagnated and motionless lifestyle is a positive spirit. In a circular manner this uplifted spirit inspires physical action that stimulates and heightens mental capacities, increases physical agility, and since it feels so good, it enlivens the spirit even more. Consequently, the individual has more reasons now to continue with an active lifestyle.

Last winter, John, an eighty year old semi-retired business person, broke both of his arms within a four month period. He continued to work in his garden despite the pain and stiffness in his arms. He stated that he had to keep moving so he would not "stiffen" up and not be able to get up again. He probably was right. Our model suggests that the circular motion becomes self-sufficient, and generates a new and healthier way of life. Although the activity may become slower with the aging years, no timekeeper exists.

There is no doubt that a variety of obstacles, both physical and psychological, contribute to the aging person's tendency to remain immobile. Most common concerns revolve around fears of falling, arthritis, stiff joints, weak muscles, and broken bones. Consequently, the older person is more inclined to favor a more sedentary lifestyle that offers little or no stimulation, less independence, and a depressed spirit. Excuses keep them house-bound. Boredom often propels them into a "couch potato" existence. Finally, the individual gains a stronger sense of uselessness and an exaggerated reminder of being old. Some individuals develop a behavioral pattern similar to learned helplessness that fuels their dependent state by generating childlike demands for any kind of attention. Nonetheless, a pattern of slow-down is often magnified and controlled by a collection of "what if" phobias.

Attitude is the secret for many older persons. According to Porterfield & Saint Pierre, the way people think and what they think can then become so.[5] For instance, if you believe illnesses and senility are inevitable in old age, then your mind has the power to generate destructive changes in your own body's physiological mechanisms. This can inevitably lead to infirmities or heightened declines.[6] Furthermore, depression can occur when older individuals think certain activities are prohibitive or restrictive, or because they believe that certain activities cannot be done at their age. These kinds of beliefs and attitudes may become self-fulfilling prophesies. Attitudes and mental depressions often lead to loss of interest. They also can lower vitality, and decrease the immune systems' defenses, therefore, a diseased or a dysfunctional state becomes predetermined by the individual's attitude. On the other hand, defeatist attitudes are unhealthy, yet, one must still maintain a healthy respect for what realistically lies within one's own control. Therefore, it means developing a balance between inevitable declines with what one can change and maintain

Many retired citizens look to the future as a time to rest and sit. Is this not like saying they look forward to declining? Furthermore, too many older persons' report that they are too old to do something because of their age. This approach may have some merit for sky-diving, but it is grossly over-stated for average daily activities. Our model suggests that the body, not the age, be the guide. This is why we recommend waltzing or light dancing and walking versus gymnastics and marathon running. If an elderly person is in comparatively good health regardless of the normal aging declines, then he or she must question their attitudes about themselves. There are two relevant questions that come to mind. First, how old would people be or feel, if they did not know how old they were? Second, how can we know how much an older person can do when few if any investigations have ever tested them to their full capabilities? We need to eliminate the stereotyped standards considered appropriate for specific ages and allow the body to be the guide, it may know more!

Walking, dancing, or simply strolling offers several positive outcomes. It keeps the elderly moving in ways analogous to our vintage cars example. It also refurbishes the person's self-image at a time of possible decline. Furthermore, it provides other avenues such as social contacts, increased appetite, elevated moods, boosted self-confidence, and most of all it keeps the "motor running." In the following chapter on exercise, the physiological benefits of keeping the motor running will be discussed. Although issues of decline will also be addressed, the advantages of walking, dancing, exercising, and continuous movement should become obvious.

Endnotes

1. Alston, S., & Silverthorne-McIntosh, S. (1991). Use it or lose it. <u>Public Health Reports, 106#2.</u> 212-213.

2. Kuhn, M., Long, C., & Quinn, L. (1991). <u>No stone unturned: The</u> life and times of Maggie Kuhn. New York: Ballantine Books.

3. Burdman, G. M. (1986). <u>Healthful aging</u>. Englewood Cliffs, NJ: Prentice Hall.

4. Cox, H. G. (1993). <u>Later life: The realities of aging,</u> (3rd ed.). Englewood Cliffs, NJ: Simon and Schuster.

5. Porterfield, J. D., & St. Pierre, R. (1992). <u>Wellness: Healthful aging.</u> Guilford, CT: Dushkin.

6. Edlin, G., & Golanty, E. (1988). <u>Health & wellness: A holistic</u> approach (3rd ed.). Boston: Jones and Bartlett

Chapter 3

Exercise Alternatives

That day the sea was green, and the sky azure blue. The white clouds were billowing specters of pearly splendor. The sun, high in the sky, radiated its golden tones. It looked unreal, somewhat like a colorful painting except for one added detail. Moving across the skyline of this panorama was a parachute resplendent in its tones of bright reds, yellows, and oranges. Eighty eight year old John was para-sailing. As he was finally lowered to the ground he shouted, "If I had known how much fun it was being old, I would have become older much sooner."

Although exercise is crucial for all ages, it can also be fun. The focus on exercise need not be a prescriptive medical must or a purposeful struggle, but simply a fundamental, animated part of life. Unfortunately, the older generation often rejects the idea of exercising in favor of a sedentary lifestyle, and feel they have earned the right to sit. Granny M. stated, "I have worked hard my whole life and looked forward to being allowed to do nothing but sit." Others, because of various rationales such as arthritis, weakened hearts, or simply retirement factors, think that this is a signal to quit and sit. Exercising work-outs are done primarily by the young and middle age groups. However, none benefits more from exercise than the elderly.[1]

It takes a certain level of psychological strength, energy and willpower to start any kind of exercise program. However, the more one works out the better one feel, and it generates the vigor and stamina needed to do more beneficial exercise. For instance, when the elderly walk infrequently, they often experience leg pain, shortness of breath, and severe fatigue. However, if they consistently carry on the physical activities, their legs feel stronger. Maintaining walking speeds with less leg pain simply requires more walking and exercise.[2] From a psychological perspective, the individual can then associate the reduced pain with consistent exercise, thus, motivating them to do more. The cumulative effect is that exercise keeps the elderly moving and fosters a more comfortable and independent lifestyle. Although numerous theories fail to explain what normal aging is, inactivity can accelerate it.[3]

According to Alston and Silverthorn-McIntosh,[4] 50% of functional decline can be attributed to disuse and excuses. Many older people believe they have already degenerated from age, and rationalize their inactivity. However, the Harvard Health Letter reports that some 70 year old athletes have pushed back their functional age by 20-25 years, therefore, it is never too late to begin an exercise program.[5] The positive effects of starting an exercise or walking series are significant and are listed as follows:

1. Increased cardiac efficiency.
2. Decreased blood pressure.
3. Slowed declines in respiratory functioning.
4. Improved nervous system functioning.
5. Improved memory.
6. Improved sleeping and other mental abilities.
7. Improved muscle strength.
8. Improved skeletal system functioning.
9. Improved endocrine system functioning.
10. Improved over-all personal feeling of well being.[6]

Furthermore, it is possible to delay or reduce many undesirable diseases or changes generated by the aging process. Although individuals who were active throughout their lifespan may show greater benefits, anyone can improve their health by exercising.

The circular interactive motion between the body, mind, and spirit becomes apparent with an exercise program and active lifestyle. DiGiovanna asserts that by incorporating consistent forms of exercise into their daily lives, the elderly can improve their cardiac output.[7] There is an element of interacting mechanistic factors with the human body. When the Cardiovascular System operations are improved, then other parts of the body function better. When this system is afflicted, however, it is analogous to a car with an impaired ignition system. The car simply runs rough. Similarly, if our Cardiovascular System is impaired, then other bodily functions may run rough. Exercise programs then can slow down physical decline and rejuvenate respiratory functioning DiGiovanna, 1994).[8] Therefore, it is easier for the individual to breath and the individual feels better.

The Muscle System is of indisputable importance with activity and exercise. Activities such as walking or other forms of exercise ease and loosen muscles and skeletal rigidity; consequently, it hurts less to move. However, there is an interesting and even more positive side to the Muscle System. DiGiovanna reports that older persons participating in a specialized exercise consistently can double their strength.[9] Furthermore, if older people participate in this type of specialized program, they can become stronger than an inactive young adult. Since muscles weakened from lack of oxygen caused by inactivity become less efficient,[10] older persons can actually increase their muscularity and improve their muscles' ability to consume oxygen simply by exercising. Furthermore, exercise stimulates mineral formation, thus, some forms of osteoporosis are prevented. Although the disease may not be fully avoided, exercise can slow down the progressive decrease in mobility, muscle mass, and fragility.[11] Muscle strength loss can reach as high as 40% by age 80, however, if an individual exercises regularly both their muscle strength and mass declines are notably reduced. Losses that do occur are experienced as gradual changes only. [12]

Too often the stigma of poor performances or possible injury deters the elderly from trying. The earlier learned habits of continual competitiveness remain with the now retired individual, and these create a psychological barrier against any active endeavors in which the individual might lose face or dignity. While race-walking one afternoon, one of the authors of this book passed an elderly gentleman who was slowly jogging. The man became incensed and stated, "you sure as hell are giving me a complex." Sadly, there was no competition, and if there had been the two would not have raced in the same age group. His feelings of intimidation most likely came from a long history of continual competitive experiences. He was feeling a sense of loss stemming from the belief that he had lost the race. Exercise for the elderly, however, is not and should not be a competitive event. It is a component in a healthy lifestyle, and a necessary ingredient for a happier life.

The exercise of choice does not have to be purposeful, but incorporated into the chosen lifestyle. For example, many elderly people avoid stairs. Although walking up stairs may be extremely difficult for an individual crippled by arthritis or degenerative diseases, a healthy older person can gain many physical benefits from using these stairs on a daily basis. The practice of avoiding chores because it takes energy and psychological strength to get out of a chair is another unproductive lifestyle pattern. The older person can incorporate some of these chores, stair walking, or simply walking each day into his or her routine life. Others might choose actual exercise plans that utilize stationary bikes, treadmills, and weights.

Older persons must move and get their bodies in motion while keeping in mind that they must perform at a level that is comfortable for their functional capacity. If it is difficult to get started, there are various warm-up activities that can be done. Maggie Kuhn's suggestion for the elderly is to use and enjoy their bubble baths.[13] Hot baths or showers do warm up the body and loosen the muscles, but care must always be taken to prevent falling. Furthermore, After an evaluation of physical limitation, a physician could recommend a start-up exercise program. However, there remains a tendency to hold the elderly back from doing certain activities when they are capable of performing them. Our model allows the individual and his body to "set the pace," meaning let your body be the guide.

A healthy older person can do much more than what the culture has designated they can do. We know now that conditions once thought of as characteristic of old age can be controlled by nutritional factors and physical exercise.[14] Most elderly fear falling, and have reservations about activities. Mobility, however, keeps the muscles stronger, and the tendency to fall becomes less. Other factors such as equilibrium problems due to medications also can be avoided. Although we will address drug issues later, the elderly must understand that mobility and activity are crucial. If their medications prevent active participation, then the drugs are possibly over-prescribed, or counter-productive. The elderly must take the reins and be in control of their own bodies. Older individuals need to discover what their bodies will do and then simply do it.

18

Endnotes

1. Improving the odds. (1991a). <u>Harvard Health Letter, 16, 4</u>.

2. Bendall, M. J., Basser, E. J., & Pearson, M. B. (1989). Factors affecting walking speed of elderly people. <u>Age and Ageing 18</u>, 327-332.

3. Cox, H. G. (1993). <u>Later life: The realities of aging</u>, (3rd ed.). Englewood Cliffs, NJ: Simon and Schuster.

4. Alston, S., & Silverthorne-McIntosh, S. (1991). Use it or lose it. <u>Public Health Reports, 106</u>, 212-213.

5. Improving the odds. (1991b). <u>Harvard Health Letter, 16, 4</u>.

6. DiGiovanna, A. G. (1994a). <u>Human aging: Biological perspectives</u> (pp. 161). New York: McGraw-Hill.

7. DiGiovanna, A. G. (1994b). <u>Human aging: Biological perspectives</u>. New York: McGraw-Hill.

8. DiGiovanna, A. G. (1994c). <u>Human aging: Biological perspectives</u>. New York: McGraw-Hill.

9. DiGiovanna, A. G. (1994d). <u>Human aging: Biological perspectives</u>. New York: McGraw-Hill.

10. Improving the odds. (1991c). <u>Harvard Health Letter, 16, 4</u>.

11. DiGiovanna, A. G. (1994e). <u>Human aging: Biological perspectives</u>. New York: McGraw-Hill.

12. Insel, P. M., & Roth, W. T. (1988). <u>Core concepts in health.</u> Palo Alto, CA: Mayfield Publishing Company.

13. Kuhn, M., Long, C., & Quinn, L. (1991). <u>No stone unturned: The life and times of Maggie Kuhn</u>. New York: Ballantine Books.

14. Porterfield, J. D., & St. Pierre, R. (1992). <u>Wellness: Healthful aging</u>. Guilford, CT: Dushkin.

Chapter 4

Learn Alternatives to Drug Therapy

There is clearly a serious epidemic of drug problems and medication issues among the elderly. Countless cases of overdosing, over-prescribing and over-usage of primarily legal drugs are widespread.[1] The elderly often see the role of physicians as drug givers, and themselves as drug takers or receivers, therefore, they expect and sometimes demand prescriptions.[2] Consequently, drugs are given to the elderly instead of alternatives that are more fitting and available. Repeatedly, prescriptions are doled out for realistic stress induced ailments that actually require social service assistance, and not a drugged state that further incapacitates the individual. Thus, the older generation often suffers from needless adverse or excessive drug effects, and their quality of life is lessened. According to Carruthers, these situations are occurring because of physician ignorance or disinterest, age-gap differences, and limited knowledge of medicinal drawbacks and non-drug alternatives.[3]

Approximately two-thirds of all prescriptions filled by the elderly are either not needed at all, unnecessarily dangerous, or dispensed with incorrect dosages.[4]. Although our model examines all three of these factors, one significant related issue that needs to be addressed is how to avoid unnecessary medications in the first place. Too often drugs are prescribed in situations for which no drug is the proper solution, such as loneliness, bereavement, or environmentally induced social isolation. For example, Seventy five year old Ruth routinely visited the doctor with numerous vague symptoms that had little disease related cause other than age. She lived in a remote country town. Her husband had died, and her children had all moved away. She had never been able to make friends easily because of her shyness, consequently, she was very lonely. Her doctor visits became a social event; yet, he occasionally misdiagnosed her symptoms, and over-prescribed drugs that were harmful to Ruth. Sometimes she became nauseous, other times too weak or lethargic to continue her chores. At one point Ruth was given Valium for emotionally induced high blood pressure. After several months of using the drug, she was dismayed to learn that she had become addicted to the Valium.

One has to question why Ruth, an educated woman with a Master's degree, would continue to use this physician. Perhaps it was because his outstanding attribute was his social skills. He would hold or pat Ruth's hand and focus with apparent interest on her complaints. Many times, he simply sat and talked to her about mundane events. When he retired, it became necessary for Ruth to find another doctor. She never liked any other physicians after him, yet, in many other ways they were more competent.

One obvious trait that Ruth seems to share with many elderly persons was her persisting tendency to hold on to the past and to use old family traditions as a bastion against personal fear and loneliness. For example, she expected her children to travel some distance to have dinner with her every Sunday although contemporary life, with its hectic and individualized lifestyles, differs radically from life fifty years ago. For many families, weekly family gatherings are simply not feasible and new ways of maintaining relationships are clearly needed. Although Ruth was physically able to visit her children by driving herself to their homes or by joining them at a restaurant, she refused to relinquish the expectations that they would come to her.

Such family traditions are a sad loss, but it does not have to mean the loss of meaningful family relationships. Ruth's own inability to accept change and adapt herself to new circumstances probably contributed to and was fueled by her growing loneliness. Instead of accepting the social challenges, she drove the car to the physician every week with numerous obscure complaints. Furthermore, by making these unnecessary visits to the doctor, she became the taker and receiver of too many drugs. More importantly, she had frequent drug reactions all because she was lonely. It would have been much better for her if she had channeled her energies into a healthier social life. Some of the drugs might have been eliminated had she not clung to the past.

Clearly, it would have been preferable for all concerned if Ruth had been able to recognize her dilemma and channel her energies into a healthier social life. Instead, her emotional reliance on her doctor probably contributed to her increasing use of drugs. Despite her intellect, she gradually lost her ability to look at matters from a new or fresh perspective and was unable to act creatively on behalf of her long-term good. Many of us, both young and old, need help with re-visioning our lives. Ill health, depression, outdated expectations, and changed circumstances can interact and pull us downward into an altered reality from which we cannot easily escape.

In an ideal world, people help one another to overcome being stuck, afraid and alone. This means reaching past inertia, stubbornness, or inconvenience when it becomes necessary to lend a helping hand by addressing fear and loneliness with compassion and hope. Ruth's physician might have seen her downward spiral and helped her to wean herself from both drugs and his attention if he had fully embraced a well ness model , like the one recommended here. Only when everyone concerned, such as family, the doctor, the American Society, friends, and Ruth herself promote wellness can situations like Ruth's find any kind of resolution.

It is difficult to make changes in one's life at any age in the lifespan, however, it is particularly arduous when one is either very young or old. There is a sense of security with old possessions and traditional habits and ways. The comfort derives from familiarity and assurance that some things will never go away. Contemporary living is far more complex and there often is not enough time for traditional rituals. Family relationships have changed dramatically as children disperse across the country to pursue their careers, and parental contact is often limited to long distance phone calls. The roles of grandparents, children and grandchildren must often be redesigned to accommodate infrequent reunions and limited cherished contacts. The elderly have had to deal with these changes while coping with other essential transformations in their lives. As their physical bodies and capabilities have been changing, their self image has also modified. Their social status is not the same and transforms dramatically if they have lost a spouse or significant loved one. Attitudinal variations in society have often challenged their moral and religious beliefs and customs. Frequently, there are too many changes for the older individual to accommodate, and it can lead to many psychological disturbances or somatic illnesses. Sometimes, it is simply loneliness; however, drugs which are too frequently prescribed do not make good company.

Our model suggests alternative strategies to drug use. For instance, a healthy lifestyle can eliminate or delay some forms of age-related degenerations and prevent some diseases from developing. We have already reported the benefits of exercise. Keep in mind, however, that any propitious results that occur from exercising will inevitably contribute to the person's well being and possibly eliminate some drug therapies.

A National Institute of Mental Health study listed seven steps for preserving one's mental health during the elderly years. All seven steps fit in with our model's assertion that some drugs can be avoided. If a person is mentally fit, their ability to cope and adapt to change is increased. An abbreviated and altered listing of the seven steps, as reported by Porterfield and St. Pierre, are:

1. Take an inventory of weaknesses and strengths. Enhance and acquire new strengths and eliminate or learn to accept the weaknesses when possible.

2. Develop and maintain a network of family and friends that can help if needed.

3. Learn to enjoy being alone. Being alone does not mean lonely. If you are comfortable with yourself, changes are easier.

4. Relax without guilt. Work might be productive, but failure to work should not inspire guilt. Other adventures should be sought.

5. Establish a weekly exercise and relaxation routine that enhances physiological, psychological, and cognitive functionings.

6. Learn to adjust to life, and whatever it brings. Power, wealth, position, and reputation are infrequently within our control, but the ability to enjoy ourselves is.

7. Accept and adapt positively to the reality of death. [5]

Other healthy lifestyle alternatives to drugs include nutritional factors and weight control. Good nutritional habits may increase one's life by as much as ten years.[6] Furthermore, they prevent many chronic ailments often associated with aging such as cancers, stroke, heart problems, diabetes, and even some psychological disorders such as depression.[7] A fat person deteriorates earlier than a slim one, therefore, obesity produces premature aging [8] Moreover, obesity and the lack of exercise has been associated with adult-onset diabetes.[9] Therefore, a nutritious diet, good weight control, and a regular exercising program might prevent the individual from having to take insulin or other diabetic medications.

One healthy alternative is to quit smoking. The obvious connection between smoking and health has been reported in cancer research. Cessation of smoking enhances one's ability to build and maintain bone matrixes, and avoid osteoporosis.[10] Too many people of all ages fail to accept the dangers of smoking and the numerous physical conditions caused by smoking. The office on Smoking and Health Centers for Disease Control reports the following types of deaths attributable to cigarette smoking:

1. Lung cancer

2. Ischemic heart disease

3. Chronic lung disease

4. Other types of cancers

5. Stroke

6. Rheumatic and pulmonary heart disease

7. Cardiac arrests

8. Hypertension

9. Atherosclerosis

10. Aortic aneurysm

11. Respiratory tuberculosis

12. Pneumonia

13. Influenza

14. Low birth rate

15. Respiratory Distress Syndrome

16. Newborn Respiratory Conditions

17. Sudden Infant Death Syndrome

18. Burn Deaths

19. Passive Smoking Deaths [11]

Looking at the variety of diseased conditions caused by cigarette smoking, the amount of health care and drug therapy used to counteract its effects should be obvious. If a person is a smoker, the only step to take toward a healthier old age is to stop smoking. Growing old does not mean that all the "good stuff" is denied. Smoking is detrimental to one's health and has no benefits at any age.

The alternative method of avoiding drug therapies is to live a healthy lifestyle. There are no guarantees that one will never have to take medicine, but a healthy lifestyle supports physical, psychological, and social well-being, and therefore, fewer drugs. Aging cannot be avoided by drugs or by lifestyle. The lifespan can be lengthened, and the quality of life enriched by productive, autonomous living. Nutrition is basic to healthful living, but individuals are products of the activity they maintain, and the habits they develop. Stringent self-denial is not necessary if moderation is incorporated into one's nutritional habits and over-indulgence is avoided. Smoking cigarettes and drinking alcohol may be immediately gratifying, but walking around with an oxygen tank or experiencing cirrhosis of the liver are not. Accepting some changes in life is a way of adapting and coping with the environment. Change that preserves options and helps promote hope and well-being over the long run deserves our embrace. Holding on to the past may be pleasant at family re-unions, but not always productive in every day life. To avoid medications, one should maximize the benefits of a social network, practice good nutrition, exercise regularly, develop a flexible mental attitude, change bad habits developed in one's youth, and find ways of cultivating gratitude. The holistic approach to wellness recommended here recognizes that both inner and outer vitality are worth cultivating and preserving, since one inevitably enhances the other.

Endnotes

1. Wolfe, S., Hope, R, & Public Citizen Health Research Group. (1993a). Worse pills best pills: The older adult's guide to avoiding drug-induced death or illness. Washington, DC: Public Citizen's Health Research Group.

   Rybash, J., Roodin, P., & Santrock, J. (1991). Adult development and aging (2nd ed.). IO: Wm C. Brown.

2. Carruthers, S. G. (1983a). Clinical pharmacology of aging. In R. D. T. Cape, R. M. Coe, & I. Rossman (Eds.). In Fundamentals of geriatric medicine, (pp. 187-196). New York: Raven Press.

3. Carruthers, S. G. (1983b). Clinical pharmacology of aging. In R. D. T. Cape, R. M. Coe, & I. Rossman (Eds.). In Fundamentals of geriatric medicine, (pp. 187-196). New York: Raven Press.

4. Wolfe, S., Hope, R, & Public Citizen Health Research Group. (1993b). Worse pills best pills: The older adult's guide to avoiding drug-induced death or illness. Washington, DC: Public Citizen's Health Research Group.

5. Porterfield, J. D., & St. Pierre, R. (1992a). Wellness: Healthful aging (pp. 104 & 106). Guilford, CT: Dushkin.

6. Porterfield, J. D., & St. Pierre, R. (1992b). Wellness: Healthful aging. Guilford, CT: Dushkin.

7. Rosenfield, I. (1985). Modern prevention: The new medicine. New York: Simon & Schuster.

8. Insel, P. M., & Roth, W. T. (1988). Core concepts in health. Palo Alto, CA: Mayfield Publishing Co.

9. Improving the odds. (1991). Harvard Health Letter, 16, 4.

10. DiGiovanna, A. G. (1994). Human aging: Biological perspectives. New York: McGraw-Hill.

11. Porterfield, J. D., & St. Pierre, R. (1992b). Wellness: Healthful aging (p. 58). Guilford, CT: Dushkin.

Chapter 5

Listen to Other Options

Listening in an active process wherein the receiver of a message must be willing to participate both mentally and physically. People tend to hear what they want to hear through selective listening. It is amazing how deaf some individuals become when the message does not agree with their own opinions or preferred way of thinking.

The processing of information requires three stages. First, reception of the message means that we have focused upon the stimulus and taken it in. In order to receive a message, we must have the physical capacity to hear it, the mental and physical capacity to pay attention, and the intellectual capacity to absorb the language. Secondly, processing the message means that we have comprehended it and added it to our filing system or memory bank. Thirdly, retrieval means that we can recall the message and bring it back to the level of consciousness for review, action, or reinterpretation. There are many theories on information processing, but we know that it is a complex chain of events, even under the best circumstances.

As we know, breakdown can occur at any stage of this process. For example, if we are upset, sick, or tired, we have a problem with focus. Further if the message is a hostile one or contrary to our commonly held beliefs, we just filter it out through selective perception. We tend to seek out those messages that agree with our commonly held beliefs, attitudes, and values. We tend to avoid those that are incongruent with our routine ways of thinking. A significant notion to remember is that all communication transactions have these two components– content or ideas, and the relationship between communicator and recipient. For example, a good friend can say things to you that are brutally honest, and you accept it in good spirit even if you do not like it. If a stranger or someone that you do not know or trust were to say the same thing, your reaction would be more defensive or even hostile. Therefore, the relationship that we have with either the sender of the message or the receiver of it is as important as the content of the message itself. Shearon Lowery and Melvin DeFleur[1] have conducted much research on selective attention, exposure, perception, and retention. These studies explain why individuals possess widely divergent psychological mechanisms which facilitate or obstruct processing information.

One of the primary roadblocks to listening is the mental barriers that we construct because we do not like the source or sender of the message. The reason for this dislike may be the history that we have with that person, or because of the many "isms" that exist, such as ageism, sexism, racism– those mental roadblocks that encourage resorting to stereotypes rather than to genuine information. If the source has credibility and we perceive that the information is relevant to us, then we are more likely to successfully receive, process, and remember the message.

There are four main causes for poor listening: not concentrating, listening too hard, jumping to conclusions, or focusing upon the delivery or personal appearances of the speakers, according to Stephen Lucas.[2]

Lack of concentration may result from boredom, fatigue, or mental confusion. Individuals tend to tune out unless they perceive that the message is important to them. Since our hearing acuity diminishes after age forty, and much sooner if one works in industrial settings or attends rock concerts, physical incapacity may make a concerted effort to hear more difficult as well. Further, people who are quite ill, mentally confused, or compromised by drugs, need an advocate or family member to run interference for them. Unfortunately, many elderly residents do not have anyone left to speak and listen for them.

<u>Listening too hard</u> sounds like a contradiction as a cause for poor comprehension; however, if the listener focuses on one word at a time rather than grasping the general meaning of the sentence, he or she may lack any understanding of what the speaker intends to convey. Listening too hard, then, involves losing the entire message by becoming stuck on a single concept or word.

A few examples may clarify the idea. Doctors frequently use polysyllabic and complex medical terminology to communicate with their patients. This may pose problems, however; for as soon as the first unfamiliar word is uttered, the listener becomes stuck trying to figure out its meaning, and ends up missing the rest of the conversation. A related difficulty arises when a single word or idea (like "cancer" or "mortality") derails the listener's information processing capacity by fostering extreme emotional distress or intense self-focus.

An added problem results when the elderly client fails to ask for clarification. Hearing difficulties, hardly uncommon among the elderly, may also complicate effective communication. Despite the fact that many elderly persons wear visible hearing aids, health care providers do not always adjust their approach by speaking more loudly, slowly, or clearly. Besides the technical vocabulary which doctors, nurses, and pharmacists use, the medical profession attracts people from all over the world. Foreign accents or dialects compound the problems in communication. Some professionals have received language tutoring and exercise care that they are understood, while others remain unintelligible even to colleagues. So failing to comprehend an important message may be attributed to physical infirmities, emotional or physical distress, and the failure of the communicator to adjust his or her message to suit the receiver's current status, vocabulary, or level of understanding.

One solution would be for the receiver to ask questions and to continue probing until the meaning of the message is clearly understood. This action requires an assertive attitude, with good self-esteem, when questioning a doctor or other professional is involved. Professionals, too, can ask questions or encourage patients to summarize what they have heard as a way of checking whether the intended message was fully received. Often patients are intimidated or afraid of appearing stupid and just passively leave the office. With all the problems in program compliance--following schedules, dietary restrictions, and behavior modification, most professionals do well to answer questions or otherwise assure patient understanding.

But many difficulties could be eliminated if both the sender and receiver of messages assume responsibility for the outcome of the communication transaction. The following suggestions would help to minimize some of the problems which occur:

Suggestions for <u>Senders</u> or <u>Speakers</u>:

1. Adjust vocabulary for the receiver. Consider educational level, experience, fears or emotional state.

2. Compensate for any mental, visual, or hearing impairment which would limit hearing or reading directions.

3. Explain the consequences for not following directions or compliance with the health care program.

4. Remember that meaning is found in receivers, not in words. Words are symbols and unless the receiver comprehends the message, no matter how learned or eloquent the speaker, the transaction is a failure. Seek common ground with the receiver.

5. Seek feedback to clarify any pitfalls or misunderstandings. Ask if the receiver has any questions.

6. Show respect for the individual regardless of age, ethnicity, income, or attitude.

Suggestions for <u>Receivers</u> or <u>Listeners</u> of Messages:

1. Pay attention and listen actively focusing upon the speaker's message.

2. Ask questions when words are unknown, directions are unclear, or concerns have not been addressed.

3. Assume responsibility to know and understand issues that will have an impact upon your life.

4. Record or make notes for future reference. A Chinese proverb says that the dullest pencil is better than the sharpest mind.

5. Respect the individual, rather than blaming them for lack of understanding, play an active role in getting the answers that you need for clarification that you seek.

If these strategies are employed then many problems can be eliminated. Another major problem with listening comes from jumping to conclusions. Closed-minded or dogmatic types of people find it difficult to admit that others actually know more about some things than they do. All listening is selective in that we must constantly filter out environmental sounds to focus on a single message. Making up one's mind about a message before the speaker can finish a sentence can have disastrous effects. One of the common ways that we jump to conclusions is by counter-arguing without listening to the speaker before we begin our debate with them. This practice results in our having held an entire argument without hearing a word the other person said. The counter-arguer interrupts others, talks louder-- mistaking volume for logic, and makes sure that he/she never has to entertain a new idea. The counter-arguer marks his exit by saying, "Yes, but..., I know, but." That "but" erases any remnants of the speaker's discourse.

Prejudicial or biased thinking results when we engage in stereotypical attitudes. Age, ethnic group, or socioeconomic status can create barriers between people. Any one of these categories can cause listeners to jump to conclusions. This writer once asked a communication class of 18 year old students, "Do you listen when people over 65 talk?" A young man said, "Well, it all depends on what they are talking about. I don't want some old man talking to me about sex." Obviously he had never heard of Masters and Johnson who are considered authorities on sexual research and were at that time three times his age.

College students consider 35 to 40 to be old. And they deny the possibility that someone over 30 could enlighten them, for example, on sexual behavior. Young people testify to the prevalence of the reverse discrimination; elders do not listen to them either, thinking that young people know little of value. Even where there is mutual respect and close friendships, each group seems to believe that the phenomena is isolated.

Another young student was required to interview two elderly individuals for a research paper in a Gerontology class. He wrote that he was amazed at his results. He found his two subjects in a local pool hall. He had thought of them before the interviews as weird old guys who wore funny clothes and argued too much about everything. After his interviews he learned that both men had been World War II heroes. Both had served together in Europe, and both had fascinating war stories to share with him. They had told him what they were doing when they were his age and he discovered something about life's cycle and how precious it is when individuals are valued for themselves.

The recent film, <u>Saving Private Ryan,</u> attests to the sacrifices and valor of that generation of young people. The popularity of that dramatic portrayal of the young soldiers in World War II with the youth in the U.S. indicates that intergenerational discourse would benefit both the young and the old. There seems to be little understanding between the generations regarding the challenges that each faces or has experienced. Some schools have organized retirees as volunteers who serve as resources to interact with students. Engineers may help students with a science project or a media person may assist students with a school event. Many serve as speakers on their areas of expertise.

In some ways the young and the old share common ground. Both groups have frequent experience with economic hardship. Both undergo identity crises involving who they may become. Both share simnilar power situations: as one group is struggling to find legitimate ways to define itself and exercise its power, the other is struggling to maintain its waning power and autonomy. Only through interaction, mutuality and good faith listening can both groups embrace the bond that draws them together, rather than feeling encumbered by it. Only by understanding their commonalities can they strive together to dispel the current of mistrust that threatens to pull them apart.

George Gerbner, Professor Emeritus from the Annenburg School of Communication, has studied the effects of mass communication for close to forty years. He has written widely and has videos on the cultivation theory of media which states that media influences the cultural environment in powerful ways. Some theories say that media has replaced the traditional institutions for teaching children values overcoming the virtues of family, religious, and educational socialization. He said that heavy viewers of television accept the images that they see of violence without consequences and of racial and gender stereotypes as more real than their actual lives. Gerbner speaks of the" mean world syndrome" where consumers of violent media images become fearful and sometimes withdrawn based upon their distorted view of reality.[3] He calls television the "electronic storyteller" which is polluting our cultural environment with imagery of violent men, women as sexual objects, and ethnic groups negatively stereotyped. The elderly are under represented or distorted in these portrayals as well. Gerbner is only one of the many scholars who have analyzed the impact of mass media upon the behavioral, attitudinal, and cognitive responses of mass consumers. He is concerned with the exposure of impressionable viewers to distorted images of the world and the impact that it is having upon the perceptions of those individuals, especially the young who are more vulnerable. We know that the social and political environment influences our views of the world and of other individuals. Elderly people are depicted as senile, powerless, or foolish. There are exceptions, like Sean Connery the actor, who continues through the decades to have romantic episodes with women one-third his age. It has been noted that we will have experienced a reality check when Sean Connery has sex with a woman his own age. Men, in mass media, are measured by their power while women are measured by their physical beauty. Clearly the distorted images that are shown repeatedly influence beliefs, attitudes, and values of viewers which are translated into their interpersonal relationships. These messages are powerful, uniform, and ubiquitous and more dangerous because of their cumulative effect. More discerning audiences can sift through the content of the "vast wasteland" as Newton Minnow, former Federal Communication Chairman in the 1960s, called television,[4] but for those who do not use the selective filters developed through maturity or learning, the impact can be devastating. The negative impact of stereotypes and distorted images can be seen as we explore the next cause for poor listening.

Focusing upon the delivery or personal appearances of the speaker is a common cause for poor listening. Sometimes the appearance of an individual alone is a cause for avoidance in communication or interaction. In the mall recently, three teenagers were hanging out wearing what most shoppers considered outlandish clothing. One young man wore combat boots, leather leggings, a vest with fringes and a spiked green Mohawk hairstyle. The other male had similar attire except that his hair was blue. The teenaged girl wore black lipstick and nail polish, an earring in both her nose and lip, a macro-mini leather skirt and a crew-cut hair style with bleached white hair. They commanded a great deal of attention in the conservatively attired community. On a bench nearby two elderly men sat talking quietly wearing plaid flannel shirts with polyester trousers and hushpuppy-type shoes. Each had a baseball cap on his head. Each group--the young teens and elderly men looked at the other as though they had just encountered a Martian. What are the chances of these two sets of individuals approaching each other to communicate? The elderly are fearful of youth violence. Deviance in dress is associated attitudinally with deviance in morals and behavior. The young are contemptuous of the pressure from elders to conform, and asserting their right to be different. The example illustrates how personal appearance can send a strong message even when no words have been uttered. We often say action speaks louder than words, but judging others as irrelevant even before they open their mouths can deny us the opportunity to truly appreciate the value of diversity and uniqueness.

Most differences are not as blatant as the example above, yet the mental barriers that we construct because of preconceived ideas about good people versus bad have the power to separate us as a society. Common expressions making use of the word "old" usually carry negative connotation, e.g., old fogey, okld snoop, old geezer, and others too colorful for this book. A 75 year old woman noted that we forgot to mention old friend, and often we need to be reminded that we have the power to assign meaning to people, events, and experiences and we need not buy into the negativism of societal labels.

The condemnation of old age and the glorification of youth have caused Americans to look upon age as a disease. As a consequence, we continue to look for the fountain of youth or clamor after miracle cures when, in fact, there is no disease but rather a natural process occurring every day--aging. This process does not begin at the moment one turns 65, but at the moment of birth. So it is not a question of whether or not we will age, unless one has the misfortune to die young, but rather the question is how we will use our time. Quality of life is the crucial issue.

The old adage that, an ounce of prevention is worth a pound of cure, applies to health at any age. Somewhere between childhood inoculations and physical education classes in public schools, we have forgotten this simple message. As individuals move along the spectrum of young adulthood, middle age, and into old age, they begin to look for a quick fix for every condition or ailment. They focus upon and listen to those messages which tell them that drug X or remedy Y will cure everything from depression to arthritis. They tune out other messages which state that they are active participants in what happens to their lives, their bodies, and their relationships with other people.

It is easier to become a passive receiver of the physician's recommendations to take a prescription than to keep a schedule to walk every day, watch food intake, and to set goals for intellectual stimulation. An 85-year old woman said, "You have to have a purpose in life and do something useful every day. This is the best time of my life." She read every day, painted landscapes when the winter made her homebound, and in spring and summer, worked in her flower and vegetable gardens. Her good fortune arose from the effort she had invested in remaining active and embracing the wellness model for living rather than embracing the medical model which would dictate that she was old and infirm and in need of medications to keep her going. She lived to be 90 surrounded by her friends and family, remaining in her own home until the last six weeks of her life when she died of lymphatic cancer. Even through the worst of times, her religious anchors gave her the stability that she required to face the unknown and to die a peaceful death.

Mass media messages bombard us with commercials for over-the-counter drugs for pain relief, digestive disorders, and irregularity. The actors in these commercials are generally older adults. The stereotypes subtly perpetuate the myth that all older people are unhealthy and need drugs. The worst effect of this media or cultural saturation is that the elderly themselves come to be indoctrinated and to believe that they fit the stereotype. Thus they feel something is wrong if they feel the urge to do youthful things like have sex, dance, go bungee jumping or parasailing. Too often they play out the frail sick role assigned to them. The messages need to change to include healthy subjects engaging in everyday pursuits into old age, and to clearly attribute the energy and joie de vivre displayed by elders to their inner strength or personal efforts, instead of to the latest medication.

Social attitudes are beginning to change as the Baby Boomers come of age in America. Recently, Robert Dole, a conservative Republican in the U.S. Senate for many years, did a commercial for Viagra, a drug prescribed for erectile dysfunction. Following the commercial, many jokes were told about Senator Dole and other older adults poking fun at any interest they might have in sex at their age. Senator Dole's willingness to address the issue of impotence indicates that attitudes are changing about medical topics that were once taboo. This incident also indicates that intimacy is something that the elderly are willing to pursue in advanced years as part of a healthy and fulfilling life. Much of the public still adheres to the stereotypes that anyone over 65 is foolish to pursue romance, much less make public statements about it. As the number of those over 65 increases, their political power base will become more vibrant with changes likely to occur.

As individuals, we may be said to have three different ages: chronological age, functional age, and psychological age. Our chronological age is determined by when we were born and how many years we have lived. Functional age is defined by how healthy or impaired our body is at any age and what we can do. Psychological age includes our maturity level. It also includes how old people feel or believe themselves to be and their attitudes, beliefs, and values regarding this age. Some 40-year olds are infirm and embittered, and conversely, some 90-year olds have ignored their chronological age to embrace life with the vitality of a child.

Attitudes toward what is appropriate and normal in old age need to change on all frontiers--in the medical community, in mass media messages, in educational institutions, and in people's self images. We have all heard the negative messages of unavoidable decline and senility and we have listened too hard to it. With repetition, the message has become ingrained, while other more positive scripts have become subordinated to the sick role.

There are other health options available to individuals besides drugs and the learned helplessness which comes from allowing others to define our lifestyle, activities, or selves. The playwright, George Bernard Shaw who lived to be 94 wrote, "The true joy of life (is) being used for a purpose recognized by yourself as a mighty one...being thoroughly worn out before you are thrown to the scrap heap...being a force of nature instead of a feverish, self clod of ailments and grievances." [5]

Shaw lived to be 94 and continued to be a powerful literary figurein old age. He was working on a new play up until his death which resulted from falling off a ladder while trimming a tree on his property at Ayot St. Lawrence in Hertfordshire.[6] A productive life, filled with ideas, and success in the theater gave him longevity and wit into his advanced years. Through his art he examined the dynamics of war, capital punishment, and other social ills. His philosophy of life was admirable and he used his years well to speak to future generations about the social conditions of his time.

His writings were radical and led to charges of treason, but his ideas live on to be re-examined by receivers who do not share the chaos of his time.

The best messages emanate from our inner voices which tell us what life means to us. Sometimes we have quieted those authentic messages to conform to the cultural scripts that others have written about us or for us. The health options that elderly individuals have open to them depend upon the combination of chronological, physical, and psychological status. In most cases, individuals' psychological orientation toward their age and physical well-being is the determining factor in motivation to engage in activities that unify the body, mind, and spirit. The circular motion mentioned earlier leads to a unified person.

Betty Friedan (1994), who wrote the <u>Fountain of Age</u>, was interviewed and quoted in <u>Parade</u> magazine. She said that as we age, we begin to see a pattern to our lives and begin to see meaning beyond the usual false dilemmas of either/or, win/lose, and zero-sum games that once obsessed us. We begin to use all that is handed to us including the pains, disasters, and surprises along with the grace notes and detours. Friedan stated that if we were willing to accept that life does not follow the pattern that we thought we were supposed to follow, then we can realize a greater freedom to enjoy all of life. We become "zestful users of serendipity" she said.[7]

Actually the pleasures of life derive neither from a fountain of youth or a fountain of age, but rather the truth of who we are as it cascades from our inner self at any given moment. Listening to our inner voice and trusting ourselves is the best of all therapies. There are distorted messages that inundate us every day reinforcing the negative images of middle age and beyond, portraying a world filled with meanness and violence. We need to take back our cultural environment by raising more reasoned discourse regarding life's special gifts of good health, friends and family, and spiritual and intellectual pursuits.

Endnotes

1. Lowery, S.A., & DeFleur, M. L. (1995). <u>Milestones in Mass Communication</u> <u>Research.</u> (3rd ed.). Needham Heights, MA: Pearson Education.

2. Lucas, S. E. (1995). <u>The art of public speaking</u>, (5th ed.). New York: Random House.

3. Black, J., & Bryant, J. (1995a). <u>Introduction to Communication.</u> (4th ed., pp.59-62). Dubuque, IA: Brown & Benchmark Publisher.

4. Black & Bryant (1995b). <u>Introduction to Communication</u>. (4th ed., pp.316-362.) Dubuque, IA: Brown & Benchmark Publisher.

5. Simpson, J. B. (1988). <u>Simpson's contemporary quotations.</u> (P. 240). Boston: Houghton Mifflin Co. 240.

6. Mazer, C.M., University of Pennsylvania. Bernard Shaw: A brief biography. Available: <u>http://www.english.upenn.edu/~cmazer/mis1.html</u>

7. Friedan, B. (1994, March 20). How to live longer, better, wiser. <u>Parade</u> <u>Magazine.</u>4-6

Chapter 6

Necessary Drugs Only

Many Americans misuse or abuse a variety of prescription, over the counter, illegal, and other un-necessary drugs. The consequences of these abusive behaviors has resulted in major drug problems for all age, race, and socioeconomic groups. Furthermore, the mass media has been a direct influence in encouraging the use of un-necessary or questionable drug use by strongly endorsing and promoting over the counter medications. In addition, it has been indirectly influential using glamorous and sophisticated advertisements that embrace alcohol consumption. However, drug abuse has been around longer than mass media advertising, thus, media promotion of various medications can be viewed as a significant influence, but not causal, so other factors are involved. The consequences of drug misuse has frequently resulted in devastated lives for people of all ages and all sectors of society. Reasons for their abusive actions have been numerous and complex.

Biological and genetic traits are two ostensible elements believed to contribute to drug-using behaviors.[1] Evidence of a genetic link has been found in some individuals that suggest a predisposition to drug abuse. For example, similar alcohol abusing behaviors have been observed in identical twins that had been separated at birth.[2] Moreover, alcoholic prone individuals show less reactions and responses to lower doses of alcohol than the nonalcoholic type indicating an inability to assess levels of intoxication. There also is evidence of different brain wave patterns in the alcoholic prone individuals that is not seen in nonalcoholics.[3] Other personality variables and attitudinal characteristics often associated with psychosocial issues have been linked with alcohol and drug abuse. Such factors as low self-esteem, antisocial behaviors, poor interpersonal skills, and developmental factors, have also been linked with alcohol abuse. Behavioral attributes, such as rebellion or a high tolerance for deviance, are frequently associated with a more positive attitude toward drugs. Payne and Associate describe several behaviors that are linked to drug use. For instance, They interpret self-indulgence in individuals as fostering feelings of pleasure. The authors reported that cigarette ads feed on that self-indulgent, pleasure principle characteristic. Escapism is another example that they proclaim as leading to drug use to promote the sense of a better life. They also maintain that individuals with poor coping skills frequently turn to drug use to help deal with the stress. Furthermore, negative childhood experiences associated with unloved and self-destructive feelings are also linked with alcohol and drug abuse. Last, environmental experiences in the home, school and community can all contribute to or influence drug abuse.[4]

The elderly may be more vulnerable to drug-use because of age-related problems. Depression is a common complaint or symptom seen in older people that could be the result of medications, social factors, and health problems. It can stem from pathological, diseased, or age-related decreases in physical activity, or be the result of learned responses, stemming from childhood, that include poor coping skills.[5] Often the reasons are more related to social problems or personal environmental stresses such as the loss of a spouse, friend, or sometimes a child. According to Crandall, bereavement, retirement, and physical illnesses are variables related to the onset of drinking alcohol.[6] However, these three factors have consequences such as depression and suicide, and there is inconclusive evidence to support whether the stressful life events precipitate alcoholism or if it is simply a relationship. Although drugs can temporarily alleviate the pain from the loss of a loved one, they cannot reverse the hurtful event. Too often the drugs only lessen the quality of life. Other options are more effective in helping the elderly cope with their losses. Therefore, if pathology is not present, consistent drug use for depression can be classified as un-necessary.

Advertising has an immense influence on both drug-use and mis-use with the elderly. Consider the countless ads from various companies that buy television and radio air time to sell their wondrous sleeping potions. This is a particularly persuasive lure for older persons who frequently have problems sleeping. According to DiGiovanna, there are several changes that occur in sleep patterns as a result of aging.[7] More time is needed to fall asleep, and frequently the elderly wake up several times during the night. Often physical conditions that include leg pains, indigestion, and arthritis will awaken them. Frequent trips to the bathroom are not uncommon. Consequently, when advertisements promise a safe and mild drug that will give them a good night's sleep, they reach for the "cure." These ads, however, fail to report many of the various side effects one can get. All drugs have multiple effects.[8] More important, no-one can be certain when side effects will occur because of the individuals' traits and lifestyle. A drug reported as safe does not apply to everyone. It refers to an average number of individuals that have positive effects when given a specific dose level. Some medication labels list the conditions when this drug is not recommended. However, a drug is not safe if it makes the person too drowsy the following day or if the "store bought drug" interferes or interacts with other medications they are taking. More important, these drugs can mask physical or emotional symptoms that require different methods of treatment.

Drug advertisements are bewitching. They are designed to attract, entice, seduce and persuade the individual into using their drugs. However, these ads are simply selling a product.[9] According to Ray & Ksir, Americans spend more than 10 billion dollars a year on over the counter products.[10] They question whether the money is spent on these drugs because of an advertising "hype" or for health issues. These are not wonder drugs, and reflect more capitalism than "medicalism." If a drug gives the individual numerous negative or unwanted side effects, then the drug is un-necessary, meaning that the bad effects outweigh the good. If drugs are used because one is simply lured by the ads for no sound purpose, then, it also is un-necessary. Beware of sub-liminal messages in ads that urge drug use. For instance, an ad might report that hay fever season is here and one should start taking a specific product. The implication is that individuals should take this drug whether they have symptoms or not.

Alcohol use is another concern for any age group, but may be particularly risky for the elderly. Many older persons have prescription drugs for age related chronic conditions, for instance high blood pressure or arthritis. Alcohol is a sedative and can relieve the pain of rigid and painful mobility. However, alcohol can cause serious interactive consequences when used with other drugs. Approximately 50% of the elderly receive anti-anxiety agents and 10-20% may receive antidepressants.[11] When alcohol is used with any tranquilizer or anti-depressants, the results can be hazardous since both have sedative effects. The mixture then is the equivalent of a double dose of a sedative.[12]

Alcohol use is a socially acceptable behavior, and our society glamorizes drinking while it also condemns it by stereotyping alcoholics as "bums or losers." These are confusing and mixed messages sent to us on alcohol use. In addition, alcohol consumption is often associated with social events. This may explain why drinking is reported as more extensive in the socially oriented retirement communities. One study indicated that 20% of retirement community residents were heavy drinkers imbibing 2 or more drinks a day.[13] Furthermore, alcohol, through obscure but collusive socializing processes, can seduce, captivate, and conquer the person. Furthermore. many individuals, from all age and socioeconomic groups are co-supporters or enablers of alcohol in social situations. These are the people whose personalities and or social positions indirectly pressure others to drink with them. These situations also strengthen the social acceptance of alcohol that is conspicuous in America. Furthermore, social confirmation reinforces denial mechanisms that often protect individuals from the reality of alcohol. When an individual secretly binges and plans binges, not only is the drinking un-necessary, it is dangerously abusive.

Moderate amounts of alcohol can promote social situations that are perceived as more positive, and aid in sleeping.[14] However, an individual should be able to have fun and socialize without the use of alcohol. When the elderly find they cannot function or socialize without the use of alcohol, then it becomes abusive and un- necessary. The necessary component for full pleasure is an experience that is not a chemically induced one.

We have become a society that turns away from unpleasant emotions seeking only gratifying experiences. Our model advises the elderly to confront all feelings and emotions rather than blur them with chemicals; reach for a friend and not a bottle. Problems are not resolved with chemical solutions nor are sound resolutions found if blurred by drugs. All people experience both joy and sorrow in life that characterizes the wide spectrum of emotions. We quickly learn that grief is the absence of joy or visa versa. Too often, while attempting to reach out or regain a sense of happiness or joy we grasp on to artificial means to lift the spirit or mood. This practice, if continued over time, eventually catches up with the person. It soon becomes apparent that the artificial means have little healing powers or abilities to resolve problems. If anything, it frequently results in the opposite effects from what the person was seeking.

The elderly have been encouraged by society in general, and physicians in particular, to become an instant-cure seeker, but often there are no cures for many of their emotional or physical ailments. Drugs can often cloud and exacerbate the problem; it becomes a co-dependent and creates stagnation. Our model supports the supposition that emotional pain over the loss of a loved one needs to be felt before the healing process can begin. For instance, when spouses die, the remaining partners are frequently left with painful feelings of loss and remorse. Unfortunately these individuals need to walk through the pain before they can get beyond it. This means they must have their period of remorse where they confront and cope with their pain. Otherwise, they may stagnate and wallow in their anguish. We believe that drugs help maintain the stagnation process by preventing the individuals from getting to the other side. Sometimes, the pain must be felt before it can get better. Unfortunately, the elderly often suffer many losses, but stagnating and wallowing in the pain delays or prevents healing or adaptation processes. A healthy life-style then for the elderly is to acquire a philosophy that minimizes drug use and maximizes living one's life thoroughly by allowing oneself to feel the wide spectrum of emotions. When you can do that, then you know you are alive.

Endnotes

1. Payne, W. A., Hahn, D. B., & Pinger, R. R.(1991a). <u>Drugs: Issues for today</u>. Baltimore: Mosby Year Book.

2. National Institute on Drug Abuse. (1988). <u>Biological vulnerability to drug abuse</u> (Research Monograph, 89). Washington, DC: U.S. Printing Office.

3. Payne, W. A., Hahn, D. B., & Pinger, R. R.(1991b). <u>Drugs: Issues for today</u>. Baltimore: Mosby Year Book.

4. Payne, W. A., Hahn, D. B., & Pinger, R. R.(1991c). <u>Drugs: Issues for today</u>. Baltimore: Mosby Year Book.

5. Porterfield, J. D., & St. Pierre, R. (1992). Wellness: <u>Healthful aging</u>. Guilford CT: Dushkin.

6. Crandall, R. C. (1991). <u>Gerontology: A behavioral science approach</u>. New York: McGraw-Hill.

7. DiGiovanna, A. G. (1994). <u>Human aging: Biological perspectives</u>. New York: McGraw-Hill.

8. Ray, O., & Ksir, C. (1993a). <u>Drugs, society, & human behavior</u>. (7th ed.) St. Louis, MO: Mosby Year Book.

9. Ray, O., & Ksir, C. (1993b). <u>Drugs, society, & human behavior</u>. (7th ed.) St. Louis, MO: Mosby Year Book.

10. Ray, O., & Ksir, C. (1993c). <u>Drugs, society, & human behavior</u>. (7th ed.) St. Louis, MO: Mosby Year Book.

11. Generations special issue on alcohol and drug abuse: Abuse and misuse. (1988a, Summer). <u>American Society on Aging</u>, 64-65.

12. Ray, O., & Ksir, C. (1993d). <u>Drugs, society, & human behavior</u>. (7th ed.) St. Louis, MO: Mosby Year Book.

13. Generations special issue on alcohol and drug abuse: Abuse and misuse. (1988b, Summer). <u>American Society on Aging</u>, 64-65.

14. Generations special issue on alcohol and drug abuse: Abuse and misuse. (1988c, Summer). <u>American Society on Aging</u>, 64-65.

Chapter 7

Eating Proper Foods–Nutrition as an Alternative to Drugs

Food is the fuel that energizes and maintains the body. Nutritional needs vary from person to person according to the individual's age, previous diseases, and current health status.

The need for good nutrition is a clear priority yet many elderly individuals are malnourished. Parker conducted a survey of 3,602 senior citizens 60 or older in December 1984 and January 1985 in 93 sites in 21 states. The data included private homes or apartments, soup kitchens, senior centers, retirement and nursing homes, shelters for homeless people, and health clinics. The group's average age was 73 years, 47.4% were low income individuals, 66.8% were women and 53.6% lived alone.[1]

Parker reported some alarming facts. He found that 18.1% of the respondents said that they did not have enough money to buy the food they needed while 38.6% said they usually had enough money to buy food and 37.6 said they always had money to purchase the food they needed. The study revealed that 5.4% had been without food for more than three days in a row in the last month of the interview while 35% ate fewer than three meals a day and 20.2% had lost weight in the last month without trying to reduce. They reflected limited variety in food selections also. He found that 9.7% had eaten less than five kinds of food the day before the interview and 21.7% of the respondents showed nutritional risks in five or more of the survey areas.

Despite these figures, food stamp participation was consistently low for the poor elderly since only 25.3% participated. The following groups said that they did not have enough food: 26.5% respondents from the soup kitchens, 20% from the food pantries, and 32.8% of those who had been without food for more than three days in a row the former month. Obviously many elderly people could use food stamps but do not.[2] Many elderly citizens are too proud to use government or state programs and some may not know that they are eligible for such support. These statistics can help professionals plan programs and mobilize community resources where they will be most useful. The consequences of malnutrition are that medical costs will inflate and individuals will suffer a diminished life.

The 29th Nestle Nutrition Workshop focused upon not just extending life, but what would be necessary to ensure quality of life.[3] The conference findings showed that the quality of life depends upon physical independence and cognitive functions. Both are influenced by the supply of proteins and carbohydrates which serve as precursors of neurotransmitters (brain chemicals) that are essential for messages to be received in the brain and carried throughout the body. There are many chronic ailments that accompany old age, but a healthy lifestyle with adequate nutrients can diminish the severity of some of the most common problems. Combating osteoporosis and osteoarthritis is secondary only to preventing obesity in the elderly population.

Virginia Newbern noted that in some cases what appears to be dementia is really malnutrition.[4] For example, Ms. C., a 68-year old retired college professor, gained weight after a couple of years of not working and began a 1,200 calorie diet and an exercise program. She played golf twice a week and swam 30 laps daily in a pool, yet she tired easily and appeared confused and paranoid at times.

Older people tend to believe that confusion and forgetfulness is a natural part of aging and that nothing can help them. They become angry, withdraw, or devise coping mechanisms like making lists to jog their memories. Ms. C. was diagnosed as having organic brain disorder of the Alzheimer's type. Actually she was suffering from a Vitamin B 12 deficiency, a condition which is reversible if caught in time. However, the condition can lead to dementia and death if not diagnosed and reversed. Other situations such as depression and hypothyroidism are sometimes misdiagnosed as dementia as well. Estimates indicate that 6.1% of people over 65 have symptoms of dementia, but one in five of these conditions can be reversed if the cause is treated according to Newbern.[5]

Studies show that dementia is not a necessary condition of old age, but rather the result of many factors. The word dementia (from the Latin de-mens, without mind) involves global deterioration of intellectual and cognitive abilities in all five major mental functions: orientation, memory, intellect, judgment, and affect.[6] Senile dementia may be reversible, irreversible and progressive. The reversible causes of dementia include:

D   Drugs

E   Emotional disorders

M   Metabolic or endocrine disorders

E   Eye and ear dysfunctions

N   Nutritional deficiencies

T   Tumor and trauma

I   Infections

A   Arteriosclerotic complications, i.e., myocardial infarction, stroke, or heart failure. [7]

The incidence of reversible dementias account for 10 to 20% while senile dementia of the Alzheimer type (SDAT) accounts for 50 to 60% of cases. Depression or pseudodementia occurs in 1 to 5%, multiple infarct dementia accounts for 20 to 30% of cases and the rest are represented by other disorders such as Parkinsons and Picks disease.[8]

It is important to remember that the majority of the elderly remain mentally competent and lucid until they die. Further, by attending to the reversible factors such as nutrition, emotional stability, and drug regiments, all of which will be discussed in further detail, we can ameliorate 10 to 20% of cases. Timiras (1994) offered statistics on dementia and he stated that severe dementia in those over 65 years can be found in only 4 to 5% and mild to moderate forms in 10%. With age however, the incidence of severe dementia increases from 0.01% at 65 to 70 to 3.5% by age 85. After 85 the incidence increases to greater than 15% among the elderly. Age is the most important risk factor for dementia in the older population[9] Nutrition is a significant factor in maintenance for all functions and prevention of complications. Age alone is not a predictor for dementia. As we noted in the foregoing causes of reversible dementia, Timiras listed nutritional deficiencies as a root cause.

Other diseases such as Diabetes type II have diet control as an essential part of the therapies applied. Henry & Edelman in 1992 discussed some of the problems associated with elderly diabetes patients.[10] Compliance to planned meals is a problem and the effect on the disease can be significant. Diet planners must take into account the individual's food preferences, ethnic background, and associated medical conditions which may also require diet restrictions. For example it is not uncommon to have an individual who has heart disease, diabetes, and arthritis. A low fat, low sodium, low sugar diet may be required for all of these combined conditions. The physician has a difficult task trying to change dietary habits that have existed for 65 years or longer. In addition, physical limitations such as visual impairment and memory loss or other functional disabilities may prevent one from getting their shopping done or food prepared as it ought to be.

Doctors Henry and Edelman concluded that every elderly patient with diabetes ought to be given a personalized plan consisting of education, dietary counseling, and an exercise plan. Walking, stationary cycling, and lap swimming are some of the most appropriate and effective forms of exercise for the elderly diabetic patient.

These benefits of dietary counseling, exercise and education ought to be a part of every individual's life. By the time one is diagnosed as having diabetes often much damage has already been done to the body. Although most elderly individuals are not overweight, 25% of elderly diabetic women aged 65 to 74 are obese, compared to 15% of women that age without diabetes. Men with diabetes have a prevalence of obesity of 6% compared to 1.5% of those without it.[11] Obesity is also a form of malnutrition. A weight loss of even five to ten pounds can produce dramatic results. Food planning and general nutrition are central issues for any healthy person. Nutrition renews, maintains, and regenerates the body.

There are many social situations that contribute to malnutrition among the elderly. In The American Dietetic Association Journal, Davis and Knutson discussed warning signals for malnutrition in the elderly.[12] Loneliness resulting from separation from one's spouse or children was a warning signal. Institutionalization, where one is left with aids or care givers, can lead to a refusal to eat. Low food intake sometimes occurs when the family is at work and the elderly members are left alone. Bereavement often leads to low food intake. Men who have lost their spouse often lack experience in dealing with food purchasing, planning, and preparation, but they are more likely to receive assistance in cooking than recently widowed women. Some less obvious causes for malnutrition included food that was given to pets rather than consumed by the owner and fad or exclusion diets.

While nutritional problems may relate to either physical or social conditions, generally they are interrelated. For example, a woman who has arthritis and is unable to go shopping for groceries without assistance may be left with few choices. Davis and Knutson concluded that conditions such as bereavement, physical or mental disabilities, and poor nutrition knowledge affect both rich and poor. [13]

Most celebrations are built around eating with our friends and family. Any change in social relationships are reflected in food consumption. The tradition of breaking bread with friends has roots throughout history and more than food is shared at a table. When one loses a spouse or friend, it is not uncommon to avoid mealtimes since they are such painful reminders of the loss. The United States Select Committee on Nutrition and Human Needs proposed that apathy and social isolation is a cause for malnutrition in the elderly because so many of our social rituals are built around eating... "therefore eating is a social and psychological event as well as a biological need."[14]

Many governmental agencies are involved in nutrition in the United States, for example, the Department of Agriculture, the Department of Health and Human Services, the U.S. Food and Drug Administration, and the National Institutes of Health. The United States Food and Drug Administration is an agency in the U.S. government that makes sure that foods are safe, wholesome, and honestly labeled along with many other functions that the agency performs such as approval of prescription and over-the-counter drugs for the public. Part of the function of the FDA is to educate the public also. In a brochure entitled, Eating Well as we Age, the FDA explored reasons that many elderly people do not eat well.[15] They offered a statement of the problems and a statement of possible solutions which are outlined below:

Problems:	Solutions:
Cannot chew	Try other foods, mashed foods, puddings, or processed foods.
Upset stomach	Try other foods.
Cannot shop	Ask for delivery, ask a family member, ask a church, synagogue, volunteer, or look for "Home Health Services" in the phone book.
Cannot cook	Cook TV dinners, participate in a group meal program-senior center, church, or meals on wheels.
No appetite	Eat with family or friends - ask doctor to review medicine. Participate in a group meal program, increase spices and herbs for flavor
Short on Money	Buy low cost foods like beans, rice, peas or pasta. Use coupons, buy on sale foods, find church or senior center, free food programs, get food stamps.

These practical hints can solve some common nutritional problems for anyone who finds themselves in the situations identified by the FDA.

In addition to the economic, physical and social factors which affect nutrition among the elderly, in the past there was disagreement among the experts over what the proper proportions or food selections ought to be. Vernon R. Young in 1990 stated that elderly people need protein allowances equal to or even greater than younger individuals and he challenged the limits set by international authorities such as the World Health Organization.[16] Young stated that with age, muscle mass diminishes, metabolism changes, and less efficient use of food results. If malnutrition occurs, the vital organs are robbed of essentials to fight stress, bacteria, or viruses, and immunological failures occur. Proteins play a key role in cell maintenance and organ function. Animal studies indicate that with age there is a reduction in tissue and organ protein synthesis along with an abnormal accumulation of enzymes which interferes with the breakdown of intercellular proteins. In humans, various theories account for the lost efficiency in body functions such as the free radical theory or error theory. Each theory postulates that as individuals age, the body and the organ systems lose their efficiency and functions break down.

Young noted that there is a progressive decline in potassium as humans age and while the significance of this process is uncertain, it usually means a loss in total body protein mass. This reduction in muscle mass appears to explain the fall in basal metabolic rate with progressing age. Amino acids such as leucine have been studied to determine their function and effects on glucose tolerance through time. Young noted that there were no major differences between younger and elderly health subjects in leucine kinetics, but it is possible that current experimental techniques fail to detect subtle deviations. Future experiments should compare leucine metabolism between age groups following stressors such as trauma or infection. Elderly individuals have limited reserves because of diminished muscle mass and reduced metabolism; thus, the immune system may be compromised. These age related declines become critical following surgery or other stresses the elderly might confront. If protein intake is insufficient then serious malnutrition results and the body's defenses are jeopardized.

In order to establish agreement in standards of nutrition which was lacking in the past, in 1999, four of the United States' top health organizations banded together to offer Unified Dietary Guidelines for nutritional protection against fatal diseases. In the past, each health agency had its own recommendations, but they have joined the American Heart Association to make it easier for the public to understand what eating right means.

A plan called the Unified Dietary Guidelines was developed by a conference of experts from the American Heart Association's Nutrition Committee with help from the American Cancer Society, American Dietetic Association, American Academy of Pediatrics, and the U.S. National Institutes of Health. The group's guidelines were published in the July 27, 1999, journal of the American Heart Association called Circulation. Richard J. Deckelbaum, M.D., co-author of the journal article, and a member of the American Heart Association Nutrition Committee, and Professor of Pediatrics and Nutrition at Columbia University said, "The good news is that we don't need one diet to prevent heart disease, another to decrease cancer risk, and yet another to prevent obesity and diabetes...A single healthy diet cuts across disease categories to lower the risk of many chronic conditions."[17]

According to the guidelines a healthy diet would include no more than 10% of calories from saturated fat, and no more than 30% from all sources of fat. Complex carbohydrates like cereal, grains, fruits and vegetables would constitute 55% of total daily calories. Cholesterol would be limited to 300 milligrams or less daily and salt would be limited to one teaspoon a day.

The Unified Dietary Guidelines were designed to meet the nutritional needs of children, women, the elderly, minorities, and the general public. These recommendations follow closely the U.S. Department of Agriculture's food pyramid. According to Edward A Fisher, a co-author of the article on behalf of the American

Heart Association and Director of lipoprotein research at New York's Mount Sinai Cardiovascular Institute in New York City, we need to eat more green, leafy vegetables that are high in antioxidants and prevent atherosclerosis which leads to heart attacks and strokes and can protect from diabetes and some forms of cancer. He said we just eat too much and obesity has skyrocketed with one-third of the United States population being significantly overweight. About 35% of American women over 20 are overweight, with Afro-American women the figure is over 50%[18]

The number of children who are overweight is growing as well. Many attribute this phenomena not only to poor nutrition, but to television which has become an addiction to some or to computer usage with games that keep children entranced and stationary for hours on end. At the same time that they are watching television or playing on the computer, they are ingesting soft drinks that are full of sugar and snacks that are empty calories as well.

The need for good nutrition is a clear priority, yet for all the reasons listed earlier–physical, social, psychological, economic, and educational, many elderly individuals are malnourished. An elderly woman once complained, "The only reason that doctors ask you everything you eat is so they can take all the things you like away from you." Individual preferences are a large part of the process too. If someone has been raised on beans and potatoes with ham hocks to flavor them, the nutritional expert will have a hard time selling brussle sprouts and summer squash as worthy competitors. Ethnicity, budget, physical and mental capacity, social contacts, and appetite are all part of the variables to be considered when we address nutrition in the elderly. Obesity may therefore be the most serious form of malnutrition in the U. S. with devastating long term effects. It increases a woman's risk for the leading causes of death–heart disease, stroke, diabetes, atherosclerosis, and cancer. A summary of the guidelines is quoted below:

Eat a variety of foods

Choose most food from plant sources

Eat five or more servings of fruits and vegetables each day.

Eat six or more servings of bread, pasta, and cereal grains each day.

Eat high fat foods sparingly, especially those from animal sources.

Keep your intake of simple sugars to a moderate level.[19]

While this panel of experts from the agencies with great research resources have reached agreement on the best diet for everyone, the controversy will continue as the public is inundated with an avalanche of high protein diets such at the Dr. Atkins' diet. Atkins has stated that obesity has increased over the years as more and more people try to follow the low fat, high carbohydrate diets. Atkins argues that the major health problems and most of our weight problems are nutritional. They arise from eating refined, processed, and devitalized food from the modern world. The culprits are not steaks and chicken breasts, Atkins says, but sugar and sweeteners, hydrogenated oils and white flour, margarine, and soda pop.[20] Others follow this train of thought with best selling books such as Sugar Busters[21] and Protein Power[22] both of which remained on the New York Times best seller's list for some time. The authors of these books, along with a legion of others, agree that refined sugar, processed grain, and too many carbohydrates are the leading causes for disease in the U.S. They maintain that obesity and diabetes did not become a problem until people began to consume large quantities of sugar. Our ancestors who had to hunt for meat and gather plants did not suffer from these diseases and the more people follow the low fat diets, they claim, the more obesity is present in the U.S. population.

The authors of the protein plans noted that the ancient Greeks and Egyptians suffered from obesity also because they enjoyed a high standard of living with diets high in grain or carbohydrates. Our early ancestors, the hunter-gatherers, had to walk miles to find game, fish, or berries to eat. Even when food sources were cultivated, the exercise one would get tending the crops and harvesting them would dictate an active lifestyle, which few Americans subscribe to today. An abundance of foods with diminished nutritional value coupled with the sedentary lifestyle of many Americans is reflected in the national crises of obesity and poor health.

February 24, 2000, the Department of Agriculture held a nutrition debate in

Washington D.C. with three of the nation's leading nutritionists and diet authors present with Dr. Barry Sears, who created the Zone diet, Dr. Robert Atkins, who has written many Atkins diet books, and Dr. Dean Ornish, who scoffed at the high-protein diets the former two promote. When the debate was over, Agriculture's Under Secretary for Food, Nutrition and Consumer Services, Shirley Watkins said, "We will stand behind the pyramid" which calls for the following:[23]

6 to 11 daily servings of pasta, bread or cereal,

2 to 3 servings of meat or other protein,

2 to 3 servings of dairy products,

2 to 4 servings of fruit,

3 to 5 servings of vegetables.

In addition to these suggestions, one should drink eight 8-ounce glasses of water a day to sustain blood pressure, prevent clots from forming or blockage of blood vessels, and to maintain kidney and bowel functions. In the debates among the various agencies or groups, water requirements are a constant recommendation. Their points of departure seem to be over how much protein or carbohydrates are required to maintain one's health.

Balanced nutrition from the beginning of one's life would prevent the diseases that occur frequently in the elderly. It would enable us to remain active and independent longer. The debate over which diet to follow will continue, but perhaps we should concede to the obvious conclusion that no diet will work alone. What is essential is healthy choices combined with portion control, nutritional foods from the different groups, and daily exercise. As research unlocks the mysteries of how each cell communicates with each other cell and enlists each system in the human body to respond to nutrients, then perhaps we will have a better understanding of how to control the diseases that diminish our lives. While food is only part of the overall picture, it is a significant part of the whole journey toward longevity and good living.

In summary, we know that many factors influence people's eating habits and these habits are resistant to change. There is hearty disagreement even among the experts on how the food groups and priorities ought to be established. The public has difficulty sifting through the quick-fix fads and the scholarly, researched recommendations. The 1999 conference among the leading health associations in the United States which created the Unified Dietary Guidelines was a step in the right direction. The debate in Washington D.C. between the different schools of thought on protein or carbohydrate dominance in a diet was also a useful dialog. Perhaps the scholarly research organizations could enlist the rhetorical skills of the writers and advocates of the fad diets so that credible information reached those who need it most.

C. Everett Koop, former Surgeon General of the U.S. during the Reagan Administration, used a public assault of information to teach the public about the AIDS epidemic over a decade ago. His campaign prioritized a topic that was taboo for some and very frightening for others with a lot of misinformation or stigma attached to it. Koop's approach broadened the debate and placed useful information in the hands of the general public in terms that could be understood. On July 20, 1998, Dr. Koop opened a Web site named Dr. Koop's Community (www.drkoop.com) where he has a forum which addresses topics such as the state of health-care coverage in the U.S., how the internet will change health-care delivery, and lifestyle factors such as smoking.[24] Koop said that he is more concerned with health care than ever before because of managed care and the state of the HMO where patients are hurried through office visits. Further with the specter of a huge aging generation, (one baby boomer turns 50 every 8.5 seconds, according to the nonprofit educational organization Population Reference Bureau.)[25], Koop sees the need for consumers to educate themselves on health issues. He was ahead of his time on the AIDS campaign, and he is ahead of most of the medical community with his website health forum. Unfortunately many without his academic background or credentials are making use of this new technology.

Obesity and malnutrition affects far more people than AIDS does in the United States. A campaign dealing with healthy diet and food selections would be useful such as the one that Koop created on AIDS during the 1980s. As noted earlier, malnutrition affects the young and old, the rich and poor alike. Individuals have an obligation to become informed on these matters, but clear guidelines with credible research behind it needs to be better communicated to those who need the help, the general public. The charlatans grow rich, while the nation grows obese with promises that pill X or Y will melt away fat while you sleep.

Nutritional counseling is a growing business where some have only name recognition or celebrity status as their primary attraction, not credentials in either medicine or nutrition. Frequently the primary function of these organizations is to sell their supplements or products to individuals who choose to believe that there is a magical solution to their obesity. We must make healthy selections, assume responsibility for our dietary habits, and when health problems arise, seek competent medical supervision for diseases that require monitoring such as arteriosclerosis, high blood pressure, diabetes, gout, arthritis, cancer and others. We identify these diseases with the elderly, but with the dietary habits of many of our young, we can expect to see a greater incidence of all of these at an earlier age.

Preventative measures would include reaching the public through health links on the internet, creating a national campaign for wellness and using mass media to share credible information to refute fad diets, and making the research findings more accessible to the general public.

Endnotes

1. Parker, S. L. (1992a). National survey of nutritional risk among the elderly. Journal of Nutrition Education, 24, 238.

2. Parker, S. L. (1992b). National survey of nutritional risk among the elderly. Journal of Nutrition Education, 24, 238.

3. Nutrition of the Elderly. (1992, January/February). Nutrition Today, 27, 33-34.

4. Newbern, V. B. (1991a). Is it really Alzheimers? American Journal of Nursing, 91, 50- 56.

5. Newbern, V .B.. (1991b) Is it really Alzheimers? American Journal of Nursing, 91, 50-56.

6. Timiras, P. S. (1994a) Aging of the nervous system: Functional changes. In P. S. Timiras (Ed.), Physiological Basis of Aging and Geriatrics. (2nd ed., pp. 103-114). Boca Raton, FL: CRC Press.

7. Timiras, P. S.(1994b) Aging of the nervous system: Functional changes. In P. S. Timiras (Ed.), Physiological Basis of Aging and Geriatrics. (2nd ed., p.108). Boca Raton, FL: CRC Press.

8. Timiras, P.S. (1994c) Aging of the nervous system: Functional changes. In P.S. Timiras (Ed.), Physiological Basis of Aging and Geriatrics. (2nd ed.). Boca Raton, FL: CRC Press.

9. Timiras, (1994d) Aging of the nervous system: Functional changes. In P.S. Timiras (Ed.), Physiological Basis of Aging and Geriatrics. (2nd ed., p. 108). Boca Raton, FL: CRC Press.

10. Henry, R. R., & Edelman, S. V. (1992a). Advances in treatment of type II diabetes mellitus in the elderly. Geriatrics, 47, 24-30.

11. Henry R. R., & Edelman, S. V. (1992b). Advances in treatment of type II diabetes mellitus in the elderly. Geriatrics, 47, 24-30.

12. Davis, L., & Knutson, K. C. (1991a). Warning signals for malnutrition in the elderly. Journal of the American Dietetic Association, 91, 1413-1417.

13. Davis L., & Knutson, K. C. (1991b), Warning signals for malnutrition in the elderly. Journal of the American Dietetic Association, 91, 1413-1417.

14. Walker, D., & Beuchene, R. E. (1991). The relationship of loneliness, social isolation, and physical health to dietary adequacy of independently living elderly. Journal of the American Dietetic Association, 91, 300.

15. U.S. Food and Drug Administration. (1999). Eating well as we age. (Publication No. 99-2311). Rockville, MD: Author.

16. Young, V. R. (1990). Amino acids and proteins in relation to the nutrition of elderly people. Age and Ageing, 19, 10-24.

17. American Heart Association.(1999a, June 22) New unified dietary guidelines offer nutritional protection against wide range of killer diseases. Available http:www.sciencedaily.com/releases/1999/06/990622061026.htm.

18. Key, S.W., & Marble, M.(1999, July 12-19) Cancer Weekly Plus, p. 15, Available: EBSCOhost. University of Pittsburgh. Item number 2034464. (CW Henderson Publisher. www.newsfile.com)

19. American Heart Association (1999b, June 22,)New unified dietary guidelines offer nutritional protection against wide range of killer diseases. Available http:www.sciencedaily.com/releases/1999/06/990622061026.htm.

20. Atkins, R. C., & Gare, F. (1997). Dr. Atkins New Diet Cookbook. New York: M. Evans and Company, Inc.

21. Steward, H. L., Bethea, M.C., Andrews, S. S., & Balart, L.A. (1998) Sugar Busters New York: Ballantine Books.

22. Eades, M.R., & Eades, D.E., (1996) Protein Power. New York: Bantam Books.

23. Rubin, A. (2000, October 10). Proper nutrition and the elderly. Available: http://www.therubins.com/aging/diet.htm.

24. Inside "Dr. Koop's Community": Q & A with C. Everett Koop. (1998a, July 22) Business Week Online. Available: http://www.businessweek.Com/bsdailydnflash'july1998/nf80722.htm.

25. Inside "Dr.Koop's Community": Q & A with C. Everett Koop (1998b, July 22) Business Week Online. Available: http://www.businessweek.Com/bsdailydnflash'july1998/nf80722e.htm.

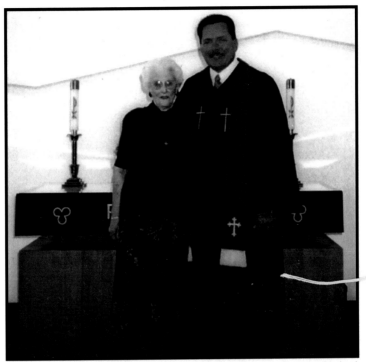

Reverend Paul Milken is pastor of the Trinity Tower United Methodist Church in Penn Hills, PA. He is also a Lieutenant Colonel in the U.S. Air Force where he has served as a chaplain for many years. Eunice Walker, 87, is a charter member of Trinity Tower and taught Sunday School for years. She has two daughters, six grandchildren, and two great-grandchildren. She is an avid traveler who organizes cultural trips for her AARP group. She still bowls and, on occasion has scored 200. Mrs. Walker has said "I have no complaints on living 87 years. I'm not anxious to go. I had a fantastic childhood, youth and marriage. My dad said, 'Get up everyday and thank the Lord for the day and don't have self-pity. Life is good.'" Some believe that folks become more religious as they age, but studies show that there is a consistency through the lifespan. Churches, synagogues, and temples are an important part of some people's lives and their gathering there keeps them connected to others in significant ways. Faith is an anchor that guides their path and comforts them when ill health, fortune, or troubles come.

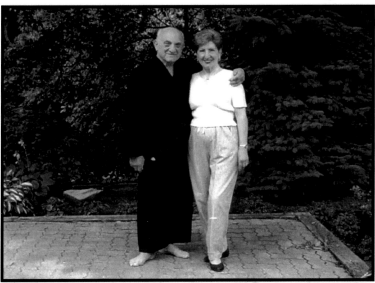

Edna Braverman, 82, is a world traveler, an avid flower gardener, and an animal lover. She is a true believer in yoga and exercise which she does daily. She has adopted four stray cats and two dogs. She and Bernie have two children, four grandchildren, and five-great grandchildren. In the neighborhood, Edna is best known for her beautiful landscaping and her Christmas decorations. Bernard Braverman, 81, is a 9th degree Black Belt in Karate. In June 2001, Bernie was inducted into the (Isshinryu, Okinawan) Hall of Fame in Gettysburg, PA. he served in the U.S. Marine Corps prior to W.W.II. Then he served in the U.S. Army for four years where he was in active combat from Africa to Germany. When Edna and Bernie married, he had a 10-day leave, but the morning after the wedding, he was called to go overseas that day. Bernie jokingly says they had the perfect marriage without a cross word for four years because they were seperated by the war like many of their generation. they have been married for 58 years.

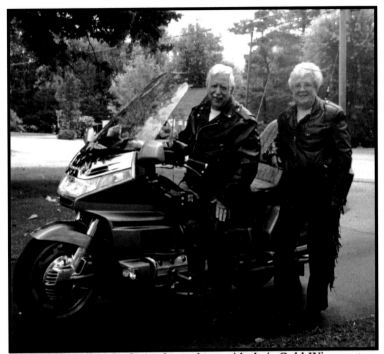

Jim and Dean Poe, both 67, shown here with their Gold Wing motorcycle, have been riding bikes since they were first married in 1952. As members of the Gold Wing Road Riders Association they participate in rallies wherein the members raise monies for charities. This year the group raised over $120,000 for the "Ride for Kids" in Marysville, Ohio, for the Pediatric Brain Tumor Foundation to further research and treatment of the children. Bikers also participate in the "Teddy Bear Ride" for the Cleveland Children's Hospital where they donate the bears to children being treated. Other activities include food banks for the needy, fund raisers for the Ronald McDonald House, and other charities. They also have road rallies just for fun.

Chapter 8

Safety and Precautionary Measures

Community and home safety is a major issue for the elderly. More than 800,000 older people are disabled every year from accidents in their homes. The effects may last a lifetime or be short term.[1]   The National Institute on Aging newsletter, Age Page, discussed accidents and the elderly. Several factors make elderly people accident prone including poor eyesight and hearing, neurological diseases, impaired coordination and balance. Many accidents can be prevented if attention is paid to safety. When accidents do occur, the elderly are most vulnerable to severe injury because they tend to heal more slowly, especially women who often have thin and brittle bones.   Various diseases, medications, alcohol and a preoccupation with personal problems can make one distracted and therefore more accident prone. Often the accidents are a manifestation of a medical condition, mental depression or poor physical conditioning.[2] People over 65 suffer 27% of all accidental deaths. The National Safety Council reports that each year 27,000 people over 65 die from accidental injuries and thousands are severely injured. Among the age group from 65 to 74, automobile accidents are the most common cause of accidental death.[3] Vehicular accidents are the second most common cause of death among older people in general. So elderly people are at risk both in their homes and on the highways of having serious accidents or being killed.

A University of Southern California survey found that some elderly people take risks that they should avoid even when they realize the danger in the situation.

The survey asked, "If the telephone were ringing and you had to cross a wet-mopped floor to answer it, would you?" About half the elderly men and women said they would not, but a third of them said they would risk crossing the wet floor to answer the telephone. Other questions on the survey concerned their perception of risks in crossing the street, bathing, and climbing stairs. Those who had experienced minor in-home accidents were more fearful of the foregoing activities and were less likely to cross the wet floor. The researchers found that there was no relationship between how risky the respondents believed the activity and the risks they were willing to take. So knowing the risk involved and choosing safety were not related.[4] The population used in the survey were out-patients at a Rehabilitation Research and Training Center on Aging in Downey, California. All of them lived independently although they were semi-frail with physical ailments resulting from arthritis, a stroke, or respiratory disease. The survey found that 20% of them said they had required medical attention for accidents which occurred at home in the last five years and 48% of them said they had been involved in a minor accident in the last year. The most frequent accident was falling.

Common causes for accidents in the home are scatter rugs that slip on the floor or trip the residents, telephone or electrical cords, broken tile, lack of bathroom railings in the shower or tub, and loose or missing handrails on steps. Some less frequent causes could be pet dishes on the floor, burners that have been turned off but remain hot, falling objects from the refrigerator or pantry shelves, and door or gate latches. It is not uncommon to see elderly persons with large bruises on their arms where door knobs or latches have bumped or torn their fragile skin. If they are taking anticoagulants, the effects are more dramatic.

In Charlottesville, VA, the Jefferson Area Board for Aging initiated a home safety program wherein a registered Occupational Therapist inspected the homes of elderly residents for safety hazards. Local government and foundation funds sponsor the program. Volunteers or paid handy men installed grab bars, built wheelchair ramps, and made other repairs for their elderly residents. The agency also showed a film on safety tips and issued a safety manual for families and professional caregivers. The program was so successful that a second video and manual were produced on sensory loss.[5]

Accidents can mean the loss of independence and require long-term care. A small investment in safety checks in homes can save medical costs and keep people out of the hospital or nursing and convalescent centers. Most people are aware of winter hazards with ice and snow, but everyday obstacles or conditions in the home are less obvious.

Sensory loss and other physical infirmities are most generally slow in development and so the impairment may not be obvious to the individual, yet they appear to others to be accident prone. Safety measures require that the elderly residents know their own limitations and pay attention to their physical environment. Bathtubs, steps, cupboard shelves and work areas that were easily negotiable once present problems as the elderly lose their range of motion, and mobility becomes compromised by arthritis, stroke, or cardio-respiratory disease. Ideally a healthy lifestyle will forestall these ill effects, but safety inspections of the home and work environment can diminish the 800,000 accidents that occur annually. Sometimes the solutions are as simple as installing lighting along driveways or steps, putting pet dishes under tables or in corners, and teaching grandchildren not to play with toys in Grandma's kitchen. Using step stools with hand bars rather than chairs to reach tall shelves could prevent many falls. Burns occur frequently when homemakers bake and touch hot racks or spill hot dishes which they may lack the strength to hold or carry safely. A man or woman living alone may continue to use the large pans, dishes, and utensils that they did when their family were living in the house. With the loss of muscle strength, lighter and smaller utensils should be used.

Old habits or routines are difficult to change. But safety awareness could be enhanced by films like the one the Jefferson County Area Board for Aging created. Workshops and seminars could be held in churches, senior centers and on television as a public service. These educational methods are useful, but are not intrusive.

It is a precarious balance to suggest different ways of doing everyday routines and yet to respect the independence of the doer. A sure way to wear out your welcome is to go into someone's home and tell them how to cook, bathe, or take care of their house. This writer did find that elderly residents were gracious and cooperative when they understood that the home visitor intended to help them to perform their daily tasks better.

A pilot program was conducted in Westmoreland County, Pennsylvania by Latrobe Area Hospital with state Agency on Aging funds.[6] The study was intended to test the effectiveness of assistive devices with 20 residents who were selected because of their in-home status and their need for help in daily routines of eating, grooming, walking, and food preparation. Four visits were made to assess their needs, to supply any helpful devices, to check on the effectiveness of the devices and to wrap up the study. The devices included special eating utensils, grab-bars for bath rooms, shampoo trays for in-bed shampoos, and other implements to help the elderly remain at home. The home visitations were quite enjoyable because we saw people coping with multiple challenges with ingenuity and great compassion most of the time. Some had already built special bed trays for eating, ramps, and other aids. Since most often women live longer than men, the frail elderly are widows without resources or skill in home maintenance. In summary, home hazards and accidents result from numerous causes:

Lack of maintenance--lack of money to repair the house, steps or walkways which create hazards for residents.

Physical debilitation of sensory capacity--diminished vision, hearing, olfactory capacity, tactile ability, and balance which are essential for self protection.

Carelessness or exercising poor judgment--crossing wet floors, leaving electrical cords on busy paths, standing on chairs to reach high places, using dim lighting for steps, driveways or garages.

Safety and precautionary measures could save elderly residents from pain and loss of life as well as control medical costs for those who must be hospitalized or treated for falls and broken bones, burns, and other preventable injuries. The goal is to keep residents in their homes living independently and enjoying life to its fullest as long as possible.

Vehicular accidents are a great concern for elderly residents as well as their families. In addition to the in-home accidents, elderly drivers over 69 are more than twice as likely to be involved in a fatal crash than those middle aged. Licensing requirements vary from state to state lack uniformity in dealing with elderly drivers. All states require vision screening, yet, the tests and their interpretation has not led to an improvement in driving assessment or safety. By the year 2000 drivers over 55 will constitute 28% of those on the roads and 30% by the year 2050.[7]

Elderly drivers are reluctant to give up their driving privileges because a driver's license symbolizes autonomy and competence not just convenience and transportation. One elderly person said. "I can barely hear, barely see, and barely walk. Things could be worse though. At least I can still drive."[8] The elderly see giving up their driver's license as a final right of passage toward immobility and dependence on others. Conversely, the young teenaged driver sees their ability to drive as a passage to freedom and independence.

According to Persson, primary causes for elderly drivers giving up their driving privileges are as follows:

> Advice from doctor
>
> Increased nervousness behind the wheel
>
> Trouble seeing pedestrians and cars
>
> Medical conditions
>
> Advice from family and friends
>
> Difficulty in coordinating hand/foot movements
>
> Cost of upkeep of vehicle or the age of vehicle
>
> Involvement in minor accident
>
> License revoked

Only 43% of participants in a study on driving said their physician had raised the topic of driving. The doctor was usually an ophthalmologist. Even fewer pharmacists (29%) had discussed the side effects of drugs while driving, and only 9% of nurses or other health care professionals like therapists discussed driving. Only 33% said family had ever raised the issue. Spouses seemed to have the most influence but most elderly drivers wanted others to "stay out of it" and allow them to make the decision. One elderly driver said, "Driving is a way of holding on to your life. I was 94 years old, and it was like losing my hand to give up driving."[9]

Drivers generally quit in two ways. The gradual approach means not driving at night or in heavy traffic, driving fewer miles, and increasing reluctance to drive with someone else in the car like their grandchildren or friends. The second approach is sudden and generally follows a disabling event like a stroke or heart attack.

Physicians should assess elderly drivers in areas of vision, reaction time and mental alertness. While many elderly live outside urban areas where public transportation is unavailable to them, the growing number of drivers over 65 will constitute a safety problem unless some uniformity in screening and control is introduced. Since driving is such a valued and essential activity, some individuals continue to operate vehicles long after it is safe for them to do so. They endanger themselves and all other people on the highway who must accommodate them.

Uniform driver tests would eliminate the incompetent drivers and sustain those who still possess the visual acuity, responses, and mental alertness to operate a vehicle. We should not assume that all drivers over 55 or 65 are incompetent. Health care professionals have been reluctant to address the issue. The lack of transportation alternatives is an important part of the dilemma. The urban elderly are better served than the rural population in public transportation. It is easier and more cost effective to serve an aggregate of people than isolated individuals who are dispersed over a large area. These rural elderly live in fear of having no public access to do banking, grocery shopping, or social activities like visiting friends or attending church. Their last line of defense is friends or family members who will drive them to medical appointments or hospitals and to other destinations essential to their continued independence. Many families are separated by great distances and unable to sustain their elderly parents. These complications have contributed to the reluctance of policy makers to come down too hard on elderly drivers who have less than perfect skills.

Elderly drivers are the butt of jokes and the source of resentment of some young drivers who bristle at their slow driving speeds or apparent ineptitude. Again, the elderly and the very young drivers share statistics as high risk operators who are most likely to have or to cause an accident. High insurance rates are one way to contain the driving hazards of both groups and these seem most uniformly applied. The young see these as discriminatory since they frequently get fines for driving too fast while the elderly do not get fines for driving too slow usually even though both extremes constitute a hazard.

In summary, standardized driving tests would eliminate those drivers who lack the capacity to operate a vehicle safely and allow those who are competent to continue their driving activities. And in-home inspections would eliminate many of the disabling accidents that elderly residents experience. Whether at home or on the road, elderly individuals who exercise good judgment concerning risk factors are more likely to remain healthy, mobile, and contented with their lives.

72

Endnotes

1. Safety program reduces risk of home accidents. (1989a). Aging, 359, 35-36

2. National Institute on Aging. Accidents and the elderly. Age Page a. U. S. Department of Health and Human Services, NIA Information Center P. O. Box - Gaithersburg, MD 20898-8057. Available: http://www.mfaa.org/center/agepage/accident_eld.html

3. National Institute on Aging. Accidents and the elderly. Age Page b. U. S. Department of Health and Human Services, NIA Information Center P. O. Box - Gaithersburg, MD 20898-8057. Available: http://www.mfaa.org/center/agepage/accident_eld.html

4. Elderly rate hazards at home. (1990, August) USA Today Newsview, 119, 2543, 12-13.

5. Safety program reduces risk of home accidents. (1989b). Aging, 239, 35-36.

6. Goldberg, J., Beeson, L. L., Darbous, P., & Getto, M. (1990). technology in personal care service. Harrisburg, PA: PA Department of Aging.

7. Persson, D. (1993a) The elderly driver: Deciding when to stop. The Gerontologist, 33. 88-91.

8. Persson, D. (1993b) The elderly driver: Deciding when to stop. The Gerontologist, 33. 88.

9. Persson, D. (1993b) The elderly driver: Deciding when to stop. The Gerontologist, 33. 90.

Chapter 9

Stress Reduction Techniques

Stress can be defined as anything that requires the organism to accommodate a change in the internal or external environment. This includes health problems, financial reversals or losses, and bad news such as the loss of a spouse or friends which produce psychic pain. As we move through life's stages into old age, we develop coping mechanisms that enable us to confront difficulties and to remain functional. In stressful situations the general adaptation mechanism has three stages according to the work of Selye conducted in the 1950s on the adrenal medulla.[1]

1. Alarm reaction. Defense mechanisms are acutely challenged.

2. State of resistance. Adaptive capacity is enhanced.

3. Stage of Exhaustion. Capacity to adapt is lost.

This model shows that our capacity to adapt is finite and can be exhausted with ongoing stress. Old age is viewed by some as accumulated stresses and strains which have confronted the individual through the lifespan. Thus, the frail elderly have low resistance to physical and psychological trauma.

It is common knowledge that impoverished people with poor nutrition, hygiene, and medical care age sooner. Prisoners of war who seem to have survived their ordeals of deprivation suffer functional impairment because of the extreme conditions they experienced. Individuals who undergo stressful conditions called the alarm reaction have stress-elevated glucocorticoids which induce catabolic reactions intended to provide energy for the emergency conditions. Selye found that these responses exact a cost to the health of the organism. He listed diabetes, hypertension, myopathy, immunosuppression, infertility, loss of weight, or inhibition of growth in children as diseases resulting from stress.[2] Continuous stress which would require secretion of adrenocordical hormones, from the thyroid, for example, or increased gluconeogenesis from protein, leads to what Selye called diseases of adaptation (atherosclerosis, gastro-duodenal ulcers, immunosuppression).

Since stress is part of living how can we manage our lives to avoid, adapt or survive the physical and psychological turmoil that bad news like loss of loved ones, financial reversals, or physical infirmities bring? The Wellness Model that we developed includes some answers:

- Develop a social network where friends or family nurture one another
- Use preventative measures to sustain the body including nutrition, daily exercise, and medical care when intervention is necessary
- Avoid cigarettes, excessive alcohol consumption, and drug dependence
- Focus on the adventures in living: love, laughter, achievements, the mysteries and spiritual dimensions of the universe

A University of Michigan Study reported by Neal Krause explored the relationship between stressful events and life satisfaction among elderly men and women.[3] The study explored the two different theories of how people view life--the bottom-up and top-down theories. The bottom-up theory states that individuals tend to compartmentalize feelings about their life. They specify certain domains or areas such as health, finances, and relationships and they synthesize these domain-specific feelings to form an overall assessment of life's satisfaction. The outcome is rather an addition of events or status to total or measure overall happiness. This view is event driven or dependent upon what is happening at a given time. The top-down theory suggests that a person's ongoing assessment of life's satisfaction is dependent upon their personal predisposition or personal interpretation of events. They tend to evaluate domain specific events in a manner that is congruent with their world view. This scenario makes the individual and their interpretation the central authority in assigning meaning to life's events. In summary, it seems that the bottoms up theory is a micro view with attention to details or specific areas and the tops down theory is a macro view with a prevailing ideology that overrides the specifics and places all of it-- health, finances, and social relationships into a perspective that is unified, balanced.

Krause offered these summary findings on how the elderly feel about life satisfaction.[4] There seem to be no consistent findings based upon age, sex, and education and life's satisfaction. Further, satisfaction with finances tend to increase with age while satisfaction with health declines. Older men are less likely to experience financial difficulty than women, but men have more chronic and debilitating diseases than women. Older people with better educations report both fewer health problems or financial problems.

If in fact research fails to point to any link between age, sex and education and reported satisfaction with life, what could the determining factor be? It would appear to be the individual's personal philosophy which explains what meaning ought to be derived from events and the coping skills that they develop through time. What one individual defines as stress another embraces as a challenge.

Bernice Cohen- Sachs made a speech at the 4th ISIS Conference in Monte Carlo, Principality of Monaco, and she said that people undergo all kinds of painful procedures in their desperate fight to stay young.[5] She mentioned having new teeth screwed into their jaws, liposuction where fat is vacuumed from their bodies, face lifts, hair transplants, breast implants for firmer bodies, penile implants for better sex, needle treatments to remove spider veins from their legs and injections of melted cow hide to smooth out their wrinkles. All of this points to a battle which uses all the weapons of modern medicine to conquer the enemy defined by our culture as old age. The trend is toward younger people having reconstructive surgery, for example, a sixteen year old having breast augmentation surgery, or women having repeated procedures done with increasing frequency.

The 74-year old speaker, Dr. Cohen-Sachs, told the session on stress management that "Old age is as much a state of mind as it is a calculation of years and an inventory of wrinkles.".[6] She told them that losses of 40 to 50% of quadriceps muscle strength which occurs between ages 20 and 60 can be reversed with a weight training program. She explained "with an appropriate exercise program, a 70-year old can increase his maximal oxygen update to the level of a sedentary 30-year old."[7] The young people who vegetate in front of television sets or computer displays are in grave danger of premature aging. Conversely, the elderly who remain active forestall the decline of muscle loss and body strength, bone thinning, and heart attacks through exercise. Physiologists have found that many symptoms of old age are the results of inactivity not the aging process. For example, studies at Duke University revealed that 70% of 68-year old men and 25% of 80-year old men had intercourse regularly if they had an interested partner.[8] Loss of erectile capacity is not a direct result of aging, but rather boredom, fatigue, medicine, fear of failure and alcohol abuse. Dr. Cohen-Sachs concluded her conference speech by saying, "I don't want to live to a good old age. I want to live a good life while I age."[9] Her conclusions on aging creatively were condensed to the following steps for coping with stress:

- exercise
- diet
- friendship
- spiritual faith and religious belief
- altruism
- compromise
- sense of humor
- self respect and dignity
- love of life
- self relaxing techniques [10]

These ideas have been addressed throughout this chapter and are enmeshed in the holistic approach to aging. We know that life's stresses produce physical illnesses. Widows and widowers have the highest incidence of cancer one year after their spouse's death than at any other time in their life.

Drug and alcohol abuse by the elderly are frequently overlooked. These problems are often the result of maladaptations to perceived stress by individuals. According to the American Encyclopedia of Drugs and Alcohol in 1995, among individuals 65 to 74, 42.5% use some amount of alcohol; only 30% do after 70. About 6% of the elderly are heavy drinkers consuming more than two drinks per day. About 5 to 12% of men and 1 to 2% of women in their 60's are problem drinkers.[11] Although drugs and drug abuse are discussed in depth elsewhere in this book, it should be noted that many alcoholics die from related causes like accidents, suicide or physical complications. A majority of male alcoholics have a strong family history of alcoholism so a genetic component is likely. Alcoholism and drug abuse lead to depression which is a primary cause for suicide.

Suicides are increasing among people over 65 according to Carpenter.. Studies focus upon three areas for research: biological theories involving physical functions, characterological theories involving personality, and cognitive theories which focus upon thought processes.[12]

Biological theories on suicide focus on biochemical and genetic causes. For instance, 60% of those who commit suicide have been identified as clinically depressed, which has a strong biochemical component. Further disruptions to brain regions like the hypothalamus and decreased neurotransmitters predispose people to impulsive acts such as suicide.

Characterological theories stress personality traits as determinants. Feelings of low self esteem or worthlessness mount from environmental factors or negative feedback propelling the individual to commit suicide to escape living with their hopelessness.

Cognitive theories on suicide concentrate on how people organize their thoughts and view the world. Suicidal individuals often engage in dichotomous thinking which means they think in opposites or dichotomies rather than in gradations. The world is seen as good or bad, pleasant or intolerable.

Despite the analytic literature on suicide, we know that more discussion on the ethics of rational suicide (meaning reasoned decisions to die when life seems no longer worth living) are occurring more frequently. Carpenter examined the arguments surrounding rational and ethical suicides in which he noted that not all suicides are linked to terminal illnesses or irrational decisions. He cited statistics that at least 2,000 to 4,000 geriatric suicides a year are not tied to pathology.[13] These individuals are free of depression, drug abuse, or cognitive impairment. This indicates that their choice shows reflection and deliberation rather than a temporary condition. Their suicides indicate a value judgment about the quality of their lives. Carpenter stated that for this category of individuals, he urges a more relaxed moral attitude toward suicide. He counter-argued against those who speak of suicide as a slippery slope to uncontrollable consequences or as the final act to cheapen the value of life. He stated that social mores somewhere along the line take a back seat to personal concerns for one who hypothetically has cardiovascular disease, arthritis, and incontinence. The slippery slope arguments includes social pressures to relieve society of the burden to sustain unproductive individuals or to relieve younger members of the care giving functions or monetary shackles that come with long term care.

These attitudes, values and beliefs about rights and responsibilities are not taken lightly. Decisions for individuals and extended families are stressful concerning the right course of treatment, the moral one, or the rational, well reasoned, one. Children of aged parents agonize over the decision to place them in nursing homes or ultimately to refuse life support measures when the loved one cannot choose for themselves. The elderly continue to live independently long after they feel assured of their capacity to do so safely, for they do not wish to be a burden to their children or society. They fight for their dignity and independence.

Euthanasia, both active and passive forms, and suicide as a reasoned decision have been put on the national agenda by Dr. Jack Kavorkian, called Dr. Death, and each of his clients. He claims that these individuals have all come to him seeking relief for their pain and suffering. They are midpoint in either a terminal illness or a life that represents so much pain that they will to end it. He claims to offer them a painless death through assisted suicide. The controversy continues about his motives, legal liabilities, and the individual's mental state who would choose to end life in such a manner.

On April 13, 1999, Jack Kevorkian, a retired pathologist was sentenced in the state of Michigan, USA, to two terms of imprisonment for helping a man with Amyotrophic Lateral Sclerosis-- Lou Gehrig's Disease, to die. He was charged with second degree murder and received a 10 to 25 year sentence; also, he received a 3 to 7 year sentence for using a lethal drug. Kevorkian had acknowledged publicly that he had assisted at least 130 people to commit suicide in the past. Other sources record fewer people involved with Kevorkian and assisted suicides, but clearly he has tested the medical profession and the U.S. courts by his actions. Thomas Youk died, with Kevorkian's help by direct injection, (active euthanasia), and when authorities failed to arrest Kevorkian, he went on the CBS television show 60 Minutes where he challenged prosecutors to act. He was arrested three days later. Kevorkian was clearly guilty of causing Tom Youk's death and the video demonstrated the drug injection. Dr. Kevorkian claimed his action did not constitute murder but was instead a justifiable act of mercy. The judge would not allow him to call Youk's wife or brother to confirm that Tom, and they, had agreed to end his suffering with the injection of a lethal drug or controlled substance.[14]

On three former occasions juries had refused to convict Kevorkian based upon the weight of the evidence. Kevorkian began to openly assist people to commit suicide in 1990. He challenged the system legally, ethically, and personally. He had his medical licenses revoked in both California and Michigan for his role in active euthanasia. There are many people who support Kevorkian in organizations such as The Euthanasia Research and Guidance Organization and the Hemlock Society USA. There are even greater numbers who fear the slippery slope that opening such a legal gateway to assisted suicide would usher into our society. They remind us of the Hippocratic oath to do no harm that physicians take and they hold to the sanctity of life as a gift that God gave to us to protect. They argue that even if a person wants to end his or her life, they have no right to expect another person to do it for them, even if they lack the physical means to do it themselves.

The age of technology has made it possible to preserve the organism even when all qualities that we identify as being uniquely human are gone – thought, communication, and personal autonomy. Kevorkian claims that suicide is a solution to end suffering and a life, determined by the possessor of it, to no longer be worth living. He will appeal his conviction and this thorny issue will not go away, even if Kevorkian is imprisoned indefinitely.

Many polls have been taken to measure support for euthanasia, but the outcome depends upon the precise question asked. In June 1997, a CNN/USA Today poll indicated 57% in favor, 35% opposed in the U.S. Three states in the U.S. have held ballot referendums with the following levels of support for euthanasia – 46% in Washington (1991), 46% in California (1992), 51% in Oregon (1994) and 60% again in Oregon (1997).[15] Like the abortion and capital punishment debates, because euthanasia is a value laden issue, the controversy will continue. It seems evident that the public is becoming more accepting of euthanasia when the person is terminally ill, especially if they are suffering, or in the process of dying rather than living a life with meaning.

The ability to adjust to the adversities of life differ greatly from individual to individual. Social and personal anchors like family and friends, a religious foundation, a strong sense of self, and a nurturing community will sustain us in the most stressful episodes. With continued stressors though, we cease to be capable of maintaining our adaptability. The Greeks long ago sought the Golden Mean with moderation in all things. We know that moderate stress can be stimulating and invigorating, but with continuing turmoil, we become ill and exhausted. The immune system is suppressed during traumatic ordeals. But medical researchers show that without mental challenges the endocrine system tends to dry up. The body, mind, and spiritual links are becoming more evident as we explore all the frontiers to being whole as human beings to the last day of our existence.

Any joyous moment that we can capture will extend life. Some individuals paint or draw, others make vegetable or flower gardens, some do volunteer work in churches, hospitals, nursing facilities, or public schools. A 98-year old music teacher serenades her friends at the Green Meadows Personal Care Community in Latrobe, PA. Her skills are so deeply ingrained that she will play the piano until her hands no longer move. The fact that she can still perform is testimony to the value of daily exercise. She keeps her identity as a performer and brings joy to her fellow residents and their families. It is the altruistic spirit which Dr. Cohen-Sachs spoke about that urges us to share love, labor, or our talents with others.

Stress reduction can derive from any activity that we enjoy, but beyond the physical or social events is the intellectual activity of challenging our minds to remain active. The mind is like a muscle--with inactivity, it degenerates. Even the frail elderly can use visualization techniques to reduce stress by returning to a favorite spot in their mind's eye. They can conjure up feelings of peace and tranquility by focusing upon a special spot like an ocean resort, their childhood hide-a-ways, or a special scene in nature. Perhaps the reason many elderly tend to live in the past is because it was a happy time. Music and art therapy are used to deflect stress or depression. The need to create or to appreciate creativity is a universal human trait.

Many elderly people express the desire to complete educational programs that were stalled by family responsibilities or disruptions like the Second World War or the Great Depression. It is a myth that the elderly cannot learn new material or skills. How well they perform depends upon the type of activity and the type of learning involved. In order to acquire knowledge, the memory must be functional. Recent studies on memory have revealed some interesting facts concerning how we learn and how age affects the learning curve. According to Timiras,[16] memory involves a three stage phenomena: processing, storage, and retrieval functions. Since the mid- 1980's studies have been conducted on the subject of aging and how memory processes work. We know that memory involves the senses of vision, hearing, touch, and smell, and an object or event to formulate a thought, the ability to store the information, and recall it later. We know that neurotransmitters are involved in memory and learning processes. We do not know which neurotransmitters or which combination of them are responsible for learning and memory. Studies reflect different neural processes for short term and long term memory. Timiras noted that:

- In sensory memory, an image is recorded very briefly, less than a second
- The information may pass on to short-term memory, which endures for several minutes
- Then to an intermediate memory to labile storage, which lasts minutes to hours, and finally
- To long term memory, which needs several hours to days to develop but which lasts a lifetime[17]

Memory loss in the elderly is restricted to short term memory while long term or intermediate memory is not affected. Therefore the myth that you can not teach old dogs new tricks is untrue. The elderly perform less well with categorizing lists but they perform well for semantic processing, association strategies, or comprehension of main points from prose material.[18] Many elderly people are avid readers and they treasure an opportunity to discuss ideas with others. Learning is not confined to the young. In order to deal with stressful situations we need to learn how to restructure our thoughts and reinterpret the meaning of events. As long as the mind is active, the elderly are capable of assigning meaning to their lives or restructuring daily events. A few have chosen to withdrawn into passivity and others have selected to escape with drugs or alcohol. The majority, however, seek mental challenge.

Biofeedback techniques exercise mind over matter to reduce pain by teaching individuals how to redirect their thoughts and responses. These areas have not been adequately appreciated in the past because of the negative expectations regarding intellectual capacity and old age.

The American lifestyle is conducive to stress related maladies such as high blood pressure, gastrointestinal complaints, depression, and heart attacks. We live by the clock and calendar of events. We cycle our sleeping, eating, and working schedules around the artificial hands of the clock rather than natural body functions and this manipulation invites disharmony or stress in everyday life. Look at the tensile like strings of headlights at 7 a.m. as the suburbanites awaken to start the trek to work and the glow of tail-lights as they return. Edward Hall in his book, The Dance of Life: The Other Dimension of Time, speaks of the cultural rhythm that propels a nation to a certain beat.[19] Hall wrote of biorhythms and cycles including those in nature. He gave examples of the Native American tribes who lived by the strokes of the seasons or the moon's phases. Somewhere in our push toward productivity and efficiency, we have lost the harmonious relationship with our own bodies and our mother earth. While we are pushed or delayed by the rest of society, we respond with internal turmoil unless we find meaningful ways to deal with our frustrations. Recent acts of violence resulting from road-rage occur on the highways triggered by some insignificant event, such as one driver cutting another off, or taking a coveted parking space, indicates that some people are out of control. The level of civility is diminished by those who believe the clock is their enemy and their schedule or plans are more important than those of others with whom they must interact. Patience is a virtue that most of us must cultivate even when we chafe under the discipline of it.

Change in our routines or condensed time lines creates stress for all of us. Retirement brings an end to the regiment known as work and the individual's synchronized patterns of existence are disrupted. For some, this lack of order, is more stressful or chaotic than the daily crush to meet deadlines, beat the clock, or survive rush hour traffic. A timely question might be a rush toward what?

Whether we appraise life from a bottoms-up view or top-down view is immaterial as long as the inventory produces feelings of satisfaction. Those individuals who have learned to manage stress, regardless of whether it is physical, social, or psychological, possess the key to longevity and personal happiness.

Endnotes

1. Timiras, P. S. (1994a). Aging of the nervous system: Functional changes. In P. S. Timiras (Ed.), Physiological Basis of Aging and Geriatrics (2nd ed., pp. 103-114). Boca Raton, FL: CRC Press.

2. Timiras, P. S. (1994b). Aging of the nervous system: Functional changes. In P. S. Timiras (Ed.), Physiological Basis of Aging and Geriatrics (2nd ed.. pp. 103-114) Boca Raton, FL: CRC Press.

3. Krause, N. (1991a). Stressful events and life satisfaction among elderly men and women. Journal of Gerontology: Social Sciences 46, 84- 92.

4. Krause, N. (1991b). Stressful events and life satisfaction among elderly men and women. Journal of Gerontology: Social Sciences 46, 84- 92.

5. Cohen-Sachs, B. (1993a January). Coping with the stress of aging creatively. Stress Magazine, 9, 45-49.

6. Cohen-Sachs, B. (1993b January). Coping with the stress of aging creatively. Stress Magazine, 9, 45.

7. Cohen-Sachs, B. (1993c January). Coping with the stress of aging creatively. Stress Magazine, 9, 46.

8. Cohen-Sachs, B. (1993d January). Coping with the stress of aging creatively. Stress Magazine, 9, 46.

9. Cohen-Sachs, B. (1993e January). Coping with the stress of aging creatively. Stress Magazine, 9, 49.

10. Cohen-Sachs, B. (1993f January). Coping with the stress of aging creatively. Stress Magazine, 9, 49.

11. Aging, drugs and alcohol. (1995) Encyclopedia of drugs and alcohol. J. H. Jaffee, (Ed.) (Vol.1, pp.51-58.) New York: Macmillan Library Reference USA.

12. Carpenter, D. (1993a). A review and new look at ethical suicide in advanced age. The Gerontologist, 33, 359-365.

13. Carpenter, D. (1993b). A review and new look at ethical suicide in advanced age. The Gerontologist, 33, 359-365.

14. Humphry, D., (2000a, November). Prisoner of conscience Dr. Jack Kevorkian, prisoner #284797 martyr to the cause of the right to choose to die. Available: http://www.finalexit.org./dr.K.html

15. Humphry, D., (2000b, November). Prisoner of conscience Dr. Jack Kevorkian, prisoner #284797 martyr to the cause of the right to choose to die. Available: http://www.finalexit.org./dr.K.html

16. Timiras, P. S. (1994c). Aging of the nervous system: Functional changes. In P. S. Timiras (Ed.), Physiological Basis of Aging and Geriatrics (2nd ed.. pp. 103-114) Boca Raton, FL: CRC Press.

17. Timiras, P. S. (1994d). Aging of the nervous system: Functional changes. In P. S. Timiras (Ed.), Physiological Basis of Aging and Geriatrics (2nd ed.. p. 107) Boca Raton, FL: CRC Press.

18. Timiras, P. S. (1994e). Aging of the nervous system: Functional changes. In P. S. Timiras (Ed.), Physiological Basis of Aging and Geriatrics (2nd ed.. p. 107) Boca Raton, FL: CRC Press.

19. Hall, E. T. (1983). The dance of life: The other dimension of time. New York Anchor Press/Doubleday.

Chapter 10

Management and Control of Drugs

Many older adults develop chronic diseases that validates the prescribing of numerous drugs, however, there is increasing evidence that countless scores of elderly take too many drugs or are over-dosed.[1] Furthermore, many diagnosed or possibly mis-diagnosed illnesses are more the results of drug interactions (prescribed or otherwise), excessive dosages of drugs, or mismanagement of the medications. Although some drug issues were reported earlier in this article and drug reactions will be addressed later, there are some principles that can help the individuals gain some control of their treatment. Self-management and control of one's medications is critical since it is one way to avoid over-medicating or over-dosing.

It is natural for people to respect and rely on the doctor's judgement, however, only the person knows his body and what he feels. According to Lindley, Tully, Paramsothy & Tallis, prescribing medications for the elderly can be problematic because of the multiple pathology commonly seen in older persons.[2] They also reported that age related changes in pharmacokinetics can lead to unpredictable plasma concentrations as well as other similar pharmacodynamics that may command more precise prescribing. Many drug reactions simply resemble symptoms of old age that are not recognized as such unless the drugs are withdrawn. Furthermore, inappropriate reporting of symptoms by the patient misleads the doctor's assessment of the problem.[3] The older person may not remember certain symptoms, or simply forget to report specific effects. Consequently, it is critical that the elderly develop a plan of action that structures the medicine taking behaviors and allows them to keep a journal on symptoms and effects. Our Wellness Model recommends the following guideline to assist the elderly in this action:

1. Make and mark a readable chart that contains times, dates, and noticeable symptoms. Each block of information per drug should include a section next to each time where the person can put an X or check-mark. In addition, there should be a journal section for notes somewhat like nurses notes on a patient's chart in a hospital. For example: if an individual is placed on a tranquilizer, he might notice that it makes him sleepy. Therefore, the chart should contain a section where notes can be made on the drug and how it affects the individual.

2. Arrange the medications in containers or paper cups with the times written on them. Then the cups should be arranged in order according to times (early to late) and kept in a large box and/or placed in a specific room.

3. Never assume you have taken a drug, and never assume that if you have forgotten to take a drug that you can simply take it later. The best approach is to develop a routine that includes charting immediately after taking the drug. If there are some questions on drugs you have forgotten to lay out or chart, or are simply not sure, it is best to check with the pharmacists. Never assume you can automatically take another drug as insurance. Also, never assume that if one pill is good, two would be better

4. Ask questions about the medications. Do not be afraid to question the doctor about any prescription, and keep a notebook on his answers. Any person as a patient has the right to know what the drug is being given for, what reactions to expect, what problems to look for, and what to do if any problems develop. If the doctor does not sufficiently answer your questions, then ask the pharmacist. In all cases you have the right to ask questions, and if you are not satisfied you have the right to ask for a second opinion. Do not be afraid to ask for literature on any drug. Some of the information may be

difficult to understand, however, adverse reactions or symptoms are generally quite clear.

5.   Generate as much interest in the cure as you have in the disease or problem. Do not automatically depend on physicians. Assuming that doctors always know best is not always the case. An individual knows himself better and longer, and should have some idea when he is being over-medicated. Read all of the literature on the drugs if available.

6.   Education on the drugs is continuous and critical. Read the literature, whenever possible, on all of the drugs. If this is not possible, then ask the doctor, nurse, or pharmacist to list the symptoms and contra-indications of the medicines' effects. Learn why the drug is prescribed. Learn what the drug is suppose to do and what the side effects are. Learn whether the drug can be addictive or habit forming. Learn whether the drug should be taken with or without food or drink, and whether certain foods are harmful. Learn whether operating any machinery or car is dangerous. Never assume that new symptoms or change in symptoms is unrelated to a specific drug, always check with the pharmacist or doctor.[4] Learn when to call the doctor with strange new symptoms that might include sleeplessness, impotency, or loss of bowel or urine control. Learn whether social drinking is safe while taking the drugs. Learn that taking someone else's prescription or over the counter-drugs might be dangerous.

90

Endnotes

1. Wolfe, S., Hope, R, & Public Citizen Health Research Group. (1993). Worse pills best pills: The older adult's guide to avoiding drug-induced death or illness. Washington, DC: Public Citizen's Health Research Group.

2. Lindley, C. M., Tully, M. P., Paramsothy, V., & Tallis, R. C. (1992). Innaproriate medication is a major cause of adverse   drug reactions in elderly patients. Age and Aging, 21, 294-300.

3. O'Neill, C. J. A., Dobbs, R. J., Dobbs, S. M., & Nicholson, P. W. (1991). Measurements of compliance with medication: The sine qua non of clinical trials in old age? Age and Ageing, 20, 77-79.

4. Folkenberg, J. (1990). Testing drugs in older people. FDA Consumer, 24, 24-27.

Chapter 11

Overcome Fears and Stereotypes Through Education

Education can be defined as Leonard did in a book called <u>Education and Ecstasy</u> on teaching philosophy as simply <u>change</u>.[1] Not all of what we learn is going to be comfortable or congruent with commonly held practices or beliefs and will require us to reorder our lifestyles and approaches to the medical community. Learning is an ongoing process from the moment of birth until death. The truly educated person continues to question basic assumptions and to seek new answers to old questions throughout life. For example, did you know that individuals over 65 compose approximately 12 percent of the population but use about 30 percent of all prescription drugs. They use about 40 percent of nonprescription drugs including sedatives and hypnotic drugs.[2] Learning includes not only facts like the former ones, but also making judgment calls about what to do with the information.

A question arises about the appropriateness of drug use or the prevalence of prescriptions for the elderly. Even though they take a disproportionate amount of drugs, should they? Maria Fiatarone, M.D. stated, "What we have in the past called aging is probably aging, plus malnutrition, plus disease."[3] She works at the Human Nutrition Research Center on aging at Tufts Research Center at Tufts University in Boston and studies muscle dysfunction and the effects of strength training in the elderly. Roy Shephard from the School of Physical and Health Education at the University of Toronto noted that whether a person is old is determined not only by chronologic age, but also by the ability to function independently. So the focus is not on pushing the limits on lifespan or extending chronologic age, but increasing the functional capacity and independence of the elderly. The New England Journal of Medicine reported that elderly men and women who used walkers increased their mobility substantially through strength training. The Hebrew Rehabilitation Center for Aged in Boston study involved 100 people, one-third of whom were in their 90s, and almost all of them had heart disease and arthritis and took multiple medications. After strength training they increased their walking speed by 12 percent and their ability to climb stairs by 28 percent. Dr. Fiatarone said that strength training can keep people from becoming chair or bed bound.[4]   Commonly stated beliefs prior to studies of this kind held that exercise could actually do harm to the frail elderly and that it should be avoided. We now know that it can mean the difference between their being able to perform the daily tasks of living such as toileting, grooming, and staying in their own homes.

Recently an exercise physiologist in a workshop this writer attended told how she works with elderly clients to enable them to maintain their strength, mobility, and independence by strength training and exercises. One 75 year-old golfer came into her center to complain that her golf game was suffering because she was losing her swing. The physiologist stated that the woman was all business, with no foolishness about her. She was very goal directed and seldom even smiled. She did follow the weight training exercises and procedures outlined at the clinic and was able to return to her prior level of functioning. First, this example illustrates that some older adults are interested in continuing sports into old age, and secondly, they expect to continue to be competitive in these endeavors. The woman knew her body well enough to know that she was losing her ability to perform as she had in the recent past. She sought a solution to her problem, and she was successful after about six weeks of training to strengthen her back and recover her range of motion and agility.

Some senior centers have incorporated weight and exercise rooms into their daily programs with special workout rooms, tread mills and weight equipment, medical staff and monitoring services. Many of these facilities resemble expensive athletic clubs, which often charge exorbitant fees, but these senior centers open the doors of opportunity to people who have never had the time or resources to belong to country clubs or athletic clubs in the past. Recently, this writer visited Center-In-The Woods, which is a senior center in California, Pennsylvania where we visited the computer room, where elders learn to surf the net, the exercise room, which was added a couple of years ago, and the dining hall, where regularly musical groups perform for the clients while they share a community meal. There are smaller spaces where community residents sit quietly and play cards, sew, or just visit. There are seminar rooms for special classes or lectures and a library. This fall, the Center-In-The-Woods will host a program which explores issues relevant to the Information Age, and will offer internet training through a program sponsored by the Pennsylvania Humanities Council called "Technology. Communication, and Community." With new words entering the lexicon like dot-com, computer virus, and e-commerce, there is a generation of people who were bypassed by computer training when it was believed that only the defense department or engineers had need of a computer. The older citizens that this writer has taught in the past in the area of technology and communication are avid learners. Many of them purchased computers right away and began networking with friends and family. Others wanted computers for very practical reasons, such as finding support groups with people who have recently had heart surgery like themselves, or to learn more about the medical conditions that they have been told that they have. Many related that their grandchildren are teaching them how to use their computer so that they can communicate via e-mail or play games with them. In these instances the technology strengthened the family and intergenerational communication.

Programs that focus upon the well elderly need to be enhanced. Many colleges and universities have non-credit courses in which those 65 and over can enroll under such organizations as elderhostel or senior initiatives without paying tuition or enjoy having reduced fees. Seniors are looking for platforms where they can share what they know with others and where they can be challenged intellectually. Some enroll in the credit courses along with the traditional students where they explore classes that they did not have time to take the first time around, or some enroll as first time college students to fulfill a dream that escaped them in their youth. Social expectations are being redefined as more people join the ranks of the over 65 generation. This flexibility in definition of jobs, learning, and family units are reconfigured to include asynchronous roles with the old being the learners and the young being the teachers sometimes.

Geriatric Education Centers, called GECS, have been developed to fill a void which existed for many years in universities and medical schools. While every stage of life was treated as a developmental speciality--Pediatrics, Adolescence, Obstetrics-Gynecology, young adulthood--the view of old age was one of decline and sickness. The geriatric model of medicine evolved out of this perceptual frame. The conventional wisdom which viewed the elderly as senile, diseased, and depressed went unchallenged for years. Medical practitioners were likely to accept confusion, the loss of muscle strength, and lack of activity or interest in life as normal aging. Further doctors would miss such diagnoses as depression, alcoholism, or sexually transmitted diseases because of prevalent images of how the elderly ought to behave or live their lives.

The Geriatric Education Centers confront the stereotypes from the past with the interdisciplinary team approach. The need to incorporate the expertise of different professionals arose from the awareness that elderly people have multiple problems and dysfunctions and that collaborative efforts were more effective in addressing the individual's needs. More importantly, the team approach included looking for strengths as well as frailty in the elderly.

One of the outcomes of the GEC training was the de-emphasis on polypharmacy, which has been a theme throughout this book. All the statistics of drug use, problems with noncompliance, pharmocokinisis, and drugs as a first line of defense were examined. Medical doctors, psychologists, social workers, nurses, and therapists began to think of changing daily routines or activities of living, to engage in psychological counseling rather than prescribing drugs, and to stress maintenance strategies for the elderly individual. Further, every elderly person was to be viewed as a resident in their home or nursing facility rather than as a patient. While this difference may be subtle linguistically, it carries a tremendous amount of weight attitudinally. To label someone as a patient means they are sick and in need of medical intervention. To call someone a resident or person means they can be treated like the rest of the population and that they require the same considerations for independence, friendship, and self determination as the normal population.

Semantics are especially significant when we know that the labels we apply to others will determine where they go, what they can do, how they are treated, and the amount of credibility they have. For example, if the physician diagnoses an elderly person as having senile dementia, the outcome is different than their having diagnosed the person as malnourished. The symptoms are sometimes the same, but malnutrition is reversible with early detection and treatment. In the first instance the individual may be moved to a nursing facility with an Alzheimer's unit and in the second instance the individual may receive some nutritional supplements and dietary guidelines and be sent home. The prevailing attitude would prejudicially focus on dementia more readily than the presence of malnourishment. The medical community, social agencies, and family members need to be aware that basic assumptions about what it means to be old must be examined in every case. More attention began to be directed to over-medication of residents as a means of social control. Protocols were established to limit the use of drugs because they were frequently seen as a means to control troublesome residents rather than as a drug essential to the individual's health status.

In 1992 there were 31 Geriatric Education Centers operating in 26 states. The funding began in 1983 from the Health Resources and Services Administration. The GECS had four educational objectives and involved multi-institutional, interdisciplinary teams of professionals to explore the various dimensions of elderly lives. Program goals were to review pharmacological issues, give specialized training to pharmacists, address medication issues for other disciplines, and to educate the public on issues relating to elderly individuals.[5]

We need to emphasize again the significance of elder drug abuse. More than 200,000 older adults are hospitalized annually for adverse drug reactions or experience them in the hospital.[6] These problems were discussed in earlier chapters along with guidelines to manage drug usage and program compliance. A survey of 72 accredited pharmacy schools in the 1985-6 school year found according to Kahl et al., "only 9 required students to take a course in geriatric pharmacy; 53 schools required minimal course content in geriatrics of 5 to 15 hours; 19 schools had no required course work in geriatrics; and 6 offered no geriatric courses at all."[7]

Let us return to the fact that we cited early in this chapter and examine what it means in the context of this discussion. Since the elderly population consume about 30 percent of all prescription medications and 40 percent of over-the-counter medications, clearly more training is essential to enable pharmacists, nurses, dentists, and others to understand the normal processes of aging and body changes that alter the way drugs are assimilated, processed, and eliminated from the body. Nurses need to know the effectiveness of the drugs prescribed and to look for adverse reactions. Half the drug therapies are written to be given as needed which leaves the nurses with major decisions on prescribing them. Dentists need to know how drugs react with elderly patients, many of whom are taking other medications as well. Social workers need to be knowledgeable so that they can refer clients who have drug-related problems to the appropriate professionals.

The elderly population themselves are in need of education on drug therapy. Noncompliance is a major problem on prescription and over-the-counter drugs. Some of the difficulties are attributable to poor memory and poor vision, but much of the problem lies in the drug culture phenomena that a quick fix is possible with drugs and if one pill is good, then two are better. Although drug reactions are addressed elsewhere, the objective of this discussion is to examine the dangers and safety issues involved. It is apparent that many problems are involved with drug use.

New technologies have been used to measure compliance with drug use in the elderly. A tablet container with a microchip memory is available to indicate opening or removal of medication. The reasoning is that if the pill box is being opened the medication is being consumed.[8] The possibility would still exist for the consumer to take more than the dose prescribed. Elderly people need to know that the more responsibility that they assume for maintaining their vitality through diet, daily exercise, and informed decision making the better their quality of life will be. An elderly woman protested when her physician called her a drug junkie that everything that she was taking was prescribed by another physician. When numerous specialists are seen to treat the elderly, it is possible for one prescription to work in contravention with another. The team approach of treatment diminishes the probability of this occurring. Drug profiles which track all the various medicines for the patient at the local pharmacy also safeguards the consumer if the pharmacist is vigilant.

Because elderly people metabolize, absorb, distribute, and excrete drugs differently, manufacturers need to determine through clinical studies what the effect of age is upon all of these functions. Judy Folkenberg offered a list of questions that elderly patients should ask their doctor or office nurse when they visit. These are found in the FDA Consumer, November, 1990 issue:[9]

- What is the drug I'm taking?
- What is the drug supposed to do?
- What are the possible side effects?
- Is the drug habit-forming?
- Should I take the drug with food or avoid food when I take it?
- Should I avoid any particular activities, such as driving a car or exercising?
- At what times of the day should I take the drug?

If elderly patients were to ask these questions, they could educate themselves on their health conditions and how the prescriptions that they are using could cause them difficulties. Many live alone or with others who are similarly frail, and they need to understand when they are in jeopardy. The relationship between doctors and their patients could be much more effective if the patient assumed responsibility for educating themselves on matters that relate to their well being directly. This requires an active approach to participating in their health plans.

Folkenberg discussed many other recommendations that the elderly could follow to ensure safety.

- Call the doctor immediately for new symptoms or side effects such as incontinence, confusion, sleeplessness or impotence
- Store medicines properly for temperature, moisture, and convenience
- Read the labels and instructions carefully
- Take the exact amount prescribed
- Do not take medicines in the dark-- turn on the light
- Flush old or expired medicines down the toilet–do not throw them away
- Do not stop taking the prescription even if you are feeling better without checking with your doctor
- Do not transfer the medicine to a different bottle
- Do not drink alcohol while you are taking medication without checking with your doctor.[10]

Wider understanding of health issues relating to the elderly needs to be nurtured both in society and in the general public themselves. Through the Geriatric Education Centers (GECs), state departments of aging, universities and social agencies, programs are being developed to look at aging not as a disease, but as a normal process. The GECS use different approaches to teach including modules offered by professionals from many fields--medical doctors, pharmacists, psychiatrists and psychologists, speech therapists and audiologists, occupational and physical therapists, nutritionists, dentists, and nurses. From their collaborative efforts, the general population and care givers have gained tremendous resource materials including research data, instructive film, pharmacy profiles, exercise programs, community based awareness efforts on smoking, alcohol, depression, sexuality, stress management, safety precautions, and bereavement.

Much is being done to address the needs of the elderly population which is increasing significantly. Until the elderly themselves become personally involved, educational programs will continue to be someone else's idea of what the elderly need and want. The best of all options is for each individual to assume responsibility for their own well being by living a healthy lifestyle. One major benefit of the educational programs is their positive thrust to repeal the negative stereotypes concerning the elderly and this is good.

100

Endnotes

1. Leonard, G. B. (1968). Education and Ecstasy. New York: Delacorte Press.

2. Kahl, A., Blandford, D. H., Krueger, K., Zwick, D.I. (1992a, January/ February). Geriatric education centers address medication issues affecting older adults. Public Health Reports. 107, 37-47.

3. Work, J.A. (1991a). Strength training: A bridge to independence for the elderly. Physician & Sports Medicine, 17 (11), 134-140.

4. Strength training helps frail elderly. Health and human development on-line magazine.Available: http://www.hhdev.psu.edu/research/Strength.htm.

5. Kahl, A., Blandford, D. H., Krueger, K., Zwick, D.I. (1992b, January/ February). Geriatric education centers address medication issues affecting older adults. Public Health Reports. 107, 37-47.

6. Kahl, A., Blandford, D. H., Krueger, K., Zwick, D.I. (1992c, January/ February). Geriatric education centers address medication issues affecting older adults. Public Health Reports. 107, 37-47.

7. Kahl, A., Blandford, D. H., Krueger, K., Zwick, D.I. (1992d, January/ February). Geriatric education centers address medication issues affecting older adults. Public Health Reports. 107, 37

8. Work, J. A. (1991b). Strength training: A bridge to independence for the elderly. Physician & Sport Medicine, 17 (11), 134-140.

9. Folkenberg, J. (November 1990a). Testing drugs in older people. FDA Consumer, 24-27.

10. Folkenberg, J. (November 1990b). Testing drugs in older people. FDA Consumer, 27.

Chapter 12

Drugs and Drug Reactions Education

The best medicine for older adults may be no medicines. Although some individuals benefit from prescription drugs for high blood pressure, arthritis, chest pain, etc., others may have extraordinary adverse effects from sensitivities to drugs (or overly prescribed drug doses) that can induce Parkinsonism, mental deterioration and confusion, and balance and coordination problems.[1] While most doctors may want their patients to know about their prescriptions, the trick is to get the older adults to ask the questions. Furthermore, patients need to be monitored once drug treatment starts, but sometimes that is not possible since communication between the elderly and physician is often faulty (preface). Therefore, older adults need a better understanding of the drugs they take, and a knowledge of the changes or symptoms to look for after they have started a new drug. Our model addressed the issue of drug literature and questions to ask in the former section. However, drugs have two sides to them, the good side and the bad. Part of the education process is learning how to recognize both sides and adequately assist the physician, as well as oneself, in assessing the efficiency and necessity of that particular drug.

According to Ray & Ksir, there are no good or bad drugs, the person who makes the choice of taking the drug determines the rightfulness of that drug.[2] Physicians also have a responsibility for the rightfulness of a prescribed medication. However, a doctor must recognize certain symptoms, and rely on the patients' complaints as the guide in determining what medications to take. He cannot predetermine all individual reactions to specific drugs, nor can he possibly know how the drugs feel unless he is given reliable information. Thus, an accurate determination and accounting of new symptoms relies on the patients' participation in their own health care. Many complaints of symptoms that resemble aging changes could be a side effect of a specific drug, or an interaction of two or more drugs. Unfortunately, the many conditions that stem from the various aging pathologies often result in polypharmacy or over-medication which is often associated with patient compliance.[3] Thus, over-prescribing of many drugs, or mis-prescribing a drug dose too strong for the elderly is common. It is crucial that physicians be informed about new symptoms that develop with new prescriptions. It is equally crucial that older adults report these changes, and that physicians pay attention to their complaints. Therefore, our model proposes that older adults must gain the knowledge and understanding of both drugs and ones' own disease process and take some control of their health.

There are several neurological problems that trigger falls in the older person, such disorders include strokes, Alzheimer's, and Parkinson's.[4] On the other hand, tranquilizers, anti-depressants, barbiturates, and some antihistamines also can increase the risk of falling. Recognizing the types or categories of drugs can be the first step in understanding their effects and interactions. For instance, tranquilizers include the better known drugs of valium (or diazepan) and librium, or the anti-depressants, prozac and elavil. Barbiturates are sedatives or sleeping pills, and antihistamines include a wide range of both prescription and over the counter drugs for colds and allergies. Some of the most common prescription drugs for high blood pressure (captopril and vasotec) can cause chest pain or angina, confusion, sleep disorders, dizziness, fainting, joint pain, numbness or tingling in hands, feet, and lips, nausea, fatigue, and urinary or bowel changes.[5] Each of these symptoms could mis-direct the physician by alluding to some other disorder or condition. However, if these symptoms develop after a new drug is started, or disappear once the drug is withdrawn, then the symptoms are probably due to the drug alone. Most people are aware of the better known drug reactions of common drugs. For instance, it is generally known that aspirin can upset the stomach. What is not commonly known is that large doses of aspirin can cause inner ear disturbances resulting in serious balance disorders and falls.

One interesting finding is that some drugs may cause conditions that are actually contra-indicated for that particular drug.[6] Although many drugs are inappropriately prescribed because of aging and related pathologies or poor presentation of the medical problem by the older patients, a great deal of the blame lies with the drug industry and the physicians.[7] The drug industry has been reported by Wolfe and Hope as inadequately testing drugs in older adults.[8] The advertising, marketing, and sale of these drugs to doctors then, contain misleading and false information about the drugs and the effects on older people. Through erroneous drug testing, that does not focus on the elderly population, implications are made that do not apply to the older adult. On the other hand, too many physicians believe that they need to write a prescription automatically following an office visit. The elderly often play into this by wanting a prescription every time they visit the doctor. One big problem is the lack of concern and interest in the elderly by many physicians. Consequently, over-prescribing and or mis-prescribing is a serious problem for older adults. According to Wolfe and Hope , there are nine reasons older adults are more likely than younger to get adverse drug reactions. These are summarized as:

- The elderly tend to weigh less, they have less water, but more proportion of fat than younger people.
- The liver does not work as well in older adults, and cannot process drugs as well as young people can.
- The kidneys in older people have a decrease in functioning ability to clear the drugs out of the body.
- The 3 other reasons listed above contribute to the elderly's greater sensitivity to many drugs.
- The blood pressure maintenance ability in the elderly changes. For instance, when a person gets out of bed the blood pressure normally

falls, decreasing the blood flow to the head. Younger individuals can compensate for that with receptors in the neck that sense that the blood pressure is falling and signal the blood vessels to tighten up in other parts of the body. Older adults receptors do not work as well, thus, they can feel giddy, light-headed, or even faint. The ability to maintain a proper blood pressure can sometimes be weakened by using some drugs (sedatives, tranquilizers, antidepressants, anti-psychotics, antihistamines, heart pain drugs, and anti-arrhythmics) causing postural hypotension and can be a leading cause of death by falls in the elderly.

- Older people do not withstand very high or low temperatures as well as young ones, and this can be worsened by several prescription and over the counter drugs. The results can be fatal or life-threatening changes in body temperatures.

- Older adults are more at risk for liver or kidney damage, poor circulation, and other chronic diseases that alter their responses to drugs.

- Older adults tend to use more prescription and over the counter drugs that greatly increases the odds of an adverse drug reaction caused by dangerous interaction between two or more drugs.

- Older people use the highest percentage of prescription drugs, yet few are adequately tested in the elderly.[9]

In some cases, simply lowering the dose may be sufficient to erase many of the problems. However, in other cases, the drug needs to be withdrawn before symptoms can be eradicated.

Not all drug reactions are serious, however, they can still cause mood changes, loss of appetite, nausea, or simply alter and diminish ones' quality of life. For instance, mood changes can often be associated with irritability, crankiness, cantankerous demeanors, and mild depressions. Although similar in nature, each of these behaviors can generate specific kinds of responses and have an enormous interactive effect with other people in the environment. National estimates of the problem of adverse drug reactions in the United States indicate a disturbing trend of drug mis-use and mis-prescribing in the elderly. For instance, 659,000 older American adults were hospitalized for adverse drug reactions in 1990. Approximately 28,000 cases of heart toxicity (adverse reaction) from digoxin result each year. Each year, approximately 41,000 older adults are hospitalized for reactions to anti-inflammatory drugs for arthritis, 3,300 die. Approximately, 9.6 million adverse drug reactions occur in older American adults. Approximately 16,000 auto crashes occur each year because of the use of psychoactive drugs by the elderly. Approximately 32,000 older American suffer from hip fractures, alone, because of drug induced fallings, at least 1500 die. One frightening finding is that 163,000 older adults in America suffer from mental impairment caused or made worse by drugs. This includes memory losses as well as dementia problems. Two million older Americans are addicted to sleeping pills or minor tranquilizers after using them daily for one year. Approximately 73,000 older Americans develop drug-induced "tardive dyskinesia" from anti-psychotic drugs. This is a condition where there is involuntary movement of the lips, tongues, and or fingers, toes, and body trunk. Last, 61,000 older Americans have developed drug induced parkinsonism because of prescribed antipsychotics.[10]

With the evidence of drug reactions now available, it is reasonable to assume that older Americans should want to take some control of their health care. Education on drug hazards should encourage the elderly to start monitoring their drug use and symptoms. Many older people fear they will either lose their mental capacities or will fall and become incapacitated. Since so many drugs induce mental impairments and hip fractures each year, the older person might consider a preventive plan. That means taking control of their drug taking behaviors, thus, becoming more responsible for their own health care.

Endnotes

1. Wolfe, S., Hope, R, & Public Citizen Health Research Group. (1993a). Worse pills best pills: The older adult's guide to avoiding drug-induced death or illness. Washington, DC: Public Citizen's Health Research Group.

2. Ray, O., & Ksir, C. (1993). Drugs, society, & human behavior. (7th ed.) St. Louis, MO: Mosby Year Book.

3. Burns, J., Sneddon, I., Lovell, M., McLean, A., & Martin, B. J. (1992). Elderly patients and their medications: A post discharge follow-up study. Age and Aging 21, 178-181.

4. Rybash, J., Roodin, P., & Santrock, J. (1991). Adult development and aging (2nd ed.).IO: Wm C. Brown.

5. Wolfe, S., Hope, R, & Public Citizen Health Research Group. (1993b). Worse pills best pills: The older adult's guide to avoiding drug-induced death or illness. Washington, DC: Public Citizen's Health Research Group.

6. Lindley, C. M., Tully, M. P., Paramsothy, V., & Tallis, R. C. (1992a). Inappropriate medication is a major cause of adverse drug reactions in elderly patients. Age and Aging, 21, 294-300.

7. Wolfe, S., Hope, R, & Public Citizen Health Research Group. (1993c). Worse pills best pills: The older adult's guide to avoiding drug-induced death or illness. Washington, DC: Public Citizen's Health Research Group. And
    Lindley, C. M., Tully, M. P., Paramsothy, V., & Tallis, R. C. (1992b). Inappropriate medication is a major cause of adverse drug reactions in elderly patients. Age and Aging, 21, 294-300. And
    O'Neill, C. J. A., Dobbs, R. J., Dobbs, S. M., & Nicholson, P. W. (1991). Measurements of compliance with medication: The sine qua non of clinical trials in old age? Age and Ageing, 20, 77-79.

8. Wolfe, S., Hope, R, & Public Citizen Health Research Group. (1993d). Worse pills best pills: The older adult's guide to avoiding drug-induced death or illness. Washington, DC: Public Citizen's Health Research Group.

9. Wolfe, S., Hope, R, & Public Citizen Health Research Group. (1993e). Worse pills best pills: The older adult's guide to avoiding drug-induced death or illness. pp. 13-16. Washington, DC: Public Citizen's Health Research Group.

10. Wolfe, S., Hope, R, & Public Citizen Health Research Group. (1993e). <u>Worse pills best pills: The older adult's guide to avoiding drug-induced death or illness</u>. pp. 10-11. Washington, DC: Public Citizen's Health Research Group.

Chapter 13

Enjoy--Have Fun and Play

The aging process is a complicated phenomena of biological, sociological, psychological, and behavioral changes that too often shapes and ascertains ones' life patterns before it is necessary.[1] Albeit, some declines will occur, but this does not necessitate an assessment of perceived inevitable and predetermined degeneration. It is too pat, and does not allow for the uniqueness and distinguishing characteristics of the human species. Although the physiological declines are unavoidable, they do not have to be predictable to the point that it predetermines the older person's behavior. This means that arthritis or stiff joints may occur, but the person is not fated to sit and do nothing the minute the symptoms begin to appear. Thus, physical, sensory, and cognitive changes do eventually occur, but the uniqueness of the human species lies in the powers of a psychological phenomena, namely the individual's attitude and other personality factors. Our model contends the powers of a positive attitude toward life, living, and aging can elevate the elderly's quality of life and challenge some physiological decrements.

Neugarten, Havighurst, and Tobin reported that more active and involved older people are more inclined to feel a greater life satisfaction.[2] Often new or role changes are adopted into their lives to keep the elderly active and involved. However, continual activity and involvement alone cannot keep the individual positive about aging nor guarantee a high level of satisfaction.[3] Not only do factors as income, health, social class, education, social supports, and interaction with others have a strong association with life satisfaction, but one's personality traits or willfulness are equally influential. Moreover, assertions by Neugarten and Bandura suggest that a sense of mastery and control over one's life is equally important.[4]

Our model questions whether our work oriented society members have lost the ability to play. Passive play is apparent with the printed media, the telephone, radio and television, but has it made the American society socially lazy? Individuals do not have to seek social encounters in an active process if they have the company of television or a telephone. However, these electronic gadgets cannot replace the interaction with friends or loved ones sharing a meal or giving you a hug. These technological advances are not as much fun as talking face to face, or playing cards with a grandchild. These wonder devices have a place and serve as some source of entertainment and in some ways combat loneliness, isolation, and stagnation. In other ways, however, they encourage more isolation through the entertainment aspects, thus, keeping the individual from making an effort to socialize. For instance, many older persons refuse social invitations because it was during the time their favorite soap opera was on. The Wellness model recognizes the importance of social systems and the active process of getting involved in life and with others. The American elderly need to enjoy the fruits of their labor and recognize that they are entitled to pleasurable experiences. Leisure and play are as essential to one's health as eating and sleeping. Fun and laughter are not restricted to the very young, and a sense of humor is cathartic and rejuvenating.

According to Cox, young children can have fun without negative connotations of idleness, sinfulness, or frivolity that often occurs when one plays in the adult years.[5] For many American adults, the values of work and commitment to work becomes a central issue in their lives. Too much free time and leisure is often associated with laziness and self-indulgence. It is difficult to change one's way of life after forty or fifty years of working. The adjustment is often abrupt, disjointing, and perplexing, and the individuals are caught off-guard and left with a pattern of role discontinuity.[6] Work has a spiritual value in America initiated by religious factors, whereas, play and leisure are associated with idleness and sinfulness. When work is no longer available, the elderly may be left with feelings of unworthiness and/or uselessness. The Puritan ethic of work is deeply ingrained in the American psyche, and the maxim "Idle hands are the Devil's workshop" still has influence.

Many elderly may argue that it is difficult to have fun, play, or seek social situations when the core of their life is gone, namely their spouses or close friends. However, contrary to the growing movement toward passive play, we are still social creatures. The process of recovering from losses such as a spouse, can be long and very depressing. Some elderly are unable to do so. Nevertheless, there are social systems and social support groups if the older people seek strength in others. Consider the following hypothetical paradigm: Marriage is frequently viewed as two people who become one. If this is true, then the loss is irreversible. If one perishes both do for the two parts have merged to become a whole unit. We need to think of marriage as two oak trees that stand side by side.[7] Their limbs wrap around each other and their roots may entangle, but they are still two entities with separate structures and systems. As the years pass, the oak trees lean toward one another frequently depending on each others strength to withstand the pressures and tensions that assault them. When death occurs to a spouse, it is analogous to the lone oak tree that has been severed from the other. Often it continues to lean toward the tree that no longer exists. Thus, it is thrown off-balance and still reaches out. One can straighten the oak tree, however, by placing supports on the other limbs of the tree and pulling it up. Like the oak tree, other support systems such as social groups and friends can buttress a person who has lost their spouse. This equalizes them and puts them back into a state of balance again.

Take the case of Grandma K, for instance, who lost her husband and two sons and with it came a despondency that rivaled clinical depression. After three months of her grieving, three friends showed up at the door demanding that she get dressed and come out with them. They told her that she had her grieving time, now it was time to get on with life. Her sense of loss was exceptional, and her life was completely off-balance, but the friends pulled her back up again. Although her life changed irrevocably, she lived another ten happy years.

The stigma of old age must first be removed. The aging process need not predict certain declines in behavior or dominate our thoughts. Second, elderly Americans need to re-evaluate the role of work. Instead of thinking they are worthless and idle they could begin by thinking that after forty years or so of working they have earned leisure time. Equally important, the social growth that develops from play for children could possibly operate as a health aid for the elderly. The older generation can have a high level of life satisfaction in play if they rid themselves of the perceived spiritual assessment of work as good and leisure as bad. Retirement should be thought of as the time to enjoy life as payback for the many years of work. It is time now to play, have fun, laugh and enjoy life. Listen to the birds you haven't heard in over sixty years.

Most elderly people have some unfinished business from their youth, unfulfilled dreams and aspirations. Countless individuals over sixty will often reflect upon the education they could not complete because of economic hardships that drove them into the work force. Others may have had musical talent that became buried under routine tasks and family obligations. Some have quieted their wonder lust to see new sights for the harness of earning a living that narrowed their horizons to a point of dullness.

The joy of learning, creative expression, and travel are not limited to the young, these are options at any age. For instance, the University of Pittsburgh has an over sixty five college, and many senior citizen groups schedule bus tours to such places as Myrtle Beach, South Carolina. When we embrace the notion that re-generativity offers life and refuse stagnation that is an existence akin to death, we then choose to rekindle the energy that drives us to the point that we enjoy every day to its fullest measure.

Although we may at times resemble the mighty oak tree that often becomes bent in a certain direction, or twisted by the wind, the oak tree is still tenacious and stately. It is the last in the forest to give up its leaves, but every spring it renews the cycle of regeneration, and so can we. Each season brings its own beauty. It behooves us to remember that we are not stuck in winter's chill even though the life cycle has been compared to the four seasons of spring, summer, fall, and winter. As a matter of fact, fall and winter bring vibrant colors and then cleansing whites. The metaphors that we choose to characterize our life are significant. The happiest people defy descriptions for they are forever in a state of renewal. None of the theories on aging can offer a blueprint for happiness because each man and woman is their own architect. Some are only dimly aware of the cathedrals that lie within their reach if they only open their minds to the potential joys that await the willing participant. It is true that some companions and sojourners will be lost along the way. It is also true, that today's complex living and societal problems can negatively influence us. However, we need to view life as a marvelous journey that has many destinations instead of perceiving death as the destination. Although death is inevitable, our destinations need to be focused on as many roads of travel as possible. Our model's prescription then is to enjoy the journey of life whatever road you travel.

Endnotes

1. Cox, H. G. (1993a). Later life: The realities of aging, (3rd ed.). Englewood Cliffs, NJ: Simon and Schuster.

2. Neugarten, B., Havighurst, R., & Tobin, S. (1968). Personality and patterns of aging. In B. Neugarten (Ed.), Middle age and aging (pp. 173-78). Chicago: University of Chicago Press.

3. Rybash, J., Roodin, P., & Santrock, J. (1991). Adult development and aging (2nd ed.). IO: Wm C. Brown.

4. Ruth, J., & Coleman P. (1996). Personality and aging: Coping and management of the self in later life. In J. E. Birren and Schaie (eds.), Handbook of the psychology of aging (pp. 308-322). New York: Van Nostrand Reinhold. And
   Bandura, A. L. (1989). Human agency in social cognitive theory. American Psychologist 44, 1175-1184.

5. Cox, H. G. (1993b). Later life: The realities of aging, (3rd ed.). Englewood Cliffs, NJ: Simon and Schuster.

6. Cox, H. G. (1993c). Later life: The realities of aging, (3rd ed.). Englewood Cliffs, NJ: Simon and Schuster.

7. Gibran, K. (1996). The Prophet. New York: Alfred A. Knopf Publisher (original work published 1923).

Chapter 14

Laughter as Internal Jogging

Laughter has been described as the best form of medicine. We were not sure why this was true for centuries, but now we know that laughter produces endorphins in the body that strengthen the immune system and produce pleasurable feelings. The field of research called psychoneuroimmunology (PNI) has established the links between the body, the mind, and the spirit as a holistic approach to life and health. Every year more studies show that your thoughts, moods, emotions, and belief system have an impact upon your body's healing mechanisms.

In this chapter, laughter will be used as a metaphor for positive emotions such as love, hope, optimism, caring, intimacy, joy, and humor. Negative emotions such as hatred, hopelessness, pessimism, indifference, anxiety, depression, and loneliness lead to illness and despair. Laughter enables people to organize their lives so that the focus is upon the positive side of the equation. This does not mean that you ignore or avoid experiencing or expressing negative emotions. Candace Pert, a former Chief of the Section on Brain Biochemistry of the Clinical Neuroscience Branch of the National Institute of Mental Health, who studied causative disease, said that in the short term, negative emotions have an enhancing effect on the immune system, but long term stress or being caught up in negativity as a habitual style, will have negative influences on your health. Pert discovered that a neuropeptide chemical messenger system connected mind and body while she was looking for specific cells in the brain where the opiate chemicals morphine and heroin are situated. Having found the brain cells to which these opiates attach themselves, she found a lock and key mechanism whereby natural chemicals fit into these receptors.[1] Further research showed that brain cells communicate with the body through neuropeptides which activates the immune and hormonal systems, and the body, in turn, communicates with the brain, activating brain cells. This circular motion demonstrates the involvement of our body, our mind, and our thoughts or feelings at a given moment. This research was only the beginning of our understanding the interactive network between the central nervous system, the autonomic nervous system, and the neuropeptide chemical messenger system. There may be other interactive systems as well. Dr Pert said, "In the beginning of my work, I matter-of-factly presumed that emotions were in the head or the brain. Now I would say they are in the body as well. They are expressed in the body and are part of the body. I can no longer make a distinction between the brain and the body.[2] We know from personal experience that when our brains are stimulated by something frightening, sad, or beautiful, that our bodies respond accordingly. The fight/flight mechanism is well known as the system that prepares us to respond in a situation that we perceive as threatening. It may be anything from giving a speech in public, taking an examination, or having a confrontation with our boss at work. Everyone knows the symptoms of rapid heartbeat, perspiration, tense muscles, and knots in the stomach. Our thoughts may be obsessed with the coming event so that more reasoned processes take a back seat. A prolonged state of readiness can exhaust us and limit our ability to respond appropriately.

Elliott S. Dacher, M.D., in the book, The New Mind/Body Healing Program, defined psychoneuroimmunology as the term that brings together the disciplines of psychology, the mind, neurology, the brain, and the immune system .[3] The impact that our thoughts have upon the body and the immune system can be demonstrated by the following example found in Dacher's book. A physician, Bruno Klopfer had a patient who was dying from cancer. When the patient heard of a miracle drug Krebiozen, he asked permission to receive it. Believing that he had only days to live, since he had received all traditional medicines, they gave him the drug. Surprisingly, the tumors shrank beyond all expectations and his vitality returned. When the same patient heard a news report saying the medicine was ineffective, the patient relapsed. The doctors then decided to give him a double dose of the medicine and again there was marked improvement and dramatic shrinking of the tumors. When a second news article noted that the drug was worthless, the patient reappeared at the hospital with a recurrence of large tumors. And he died several days later.[4] Dasher concluded, "The brain appears to play the central administrative role in translating the content of the mind, attitude, and perceptions, into nerve impulses and biochemistry. It then communicates with the body through the nervous system, consisting of nerves extending from the brain to the remainder of the body and biochemicals that circulate through the body"[5] Therefore our thoughts, feelings, sensations, and images affect our health and well being. Dasher showed how the immune cells identify and destroy bacteria, viruses, and abnormal cells, heal wounds, and maintain homeostasis. Neuropeptides and hormonal cells release hormones, activate physiology and maintain homeostasis. When stress is ongoing and there is no relaxation from it to allow emotional well-being, then individuals become ill. Dasher showed how job strains, loneliness, and loss can lead to illness. He cited two studies to support his conclusions. Peter L. Schnall, M.D. and colleagues reported in the Journal of American Medical Association that individuals with job strain have a three-times higher risk of developing high blood pressure and increased incidence of structural damage to the heart. They based their findings upon a sample of 215 men. Steven Schleiffer and colleagues at Mount Sinai School of Medicine in New York City found detectable suppression of the immune system during the bereavement period of men who had recently lost their wives. Several studies show a higher incidence of infectious disease, heart disease, and cancer associated with marital divorce and separation.[6] Bad marriages or relationships can lead to associated biochemical changes including immune suppression, ulcerative colitis, and other systemic diseases. Dasher recommends self-healing through self-directed change.

He said we can use the mind which has two operating systems: mind-talk and mindfulness. Mind-talk includes thoughts, feelings, images and sensations and is characterized by scattered thinking, a restless mind, and an activated body. The sources of mind-talk are memories and current events. Mindfulness includes attention, concentration, and meditation which are characterized by focused awareness, a quiet mind, and a still body. The sources of mindfulness are found in present moments which requires controlling the rambling chaotic mind of mind-talk. In order to achieve mindfulness, one must have three things: a positive attitude, solitude to think, reflect, and concentrate upon the processes that evoke discomfort or stress in one's life, and patience.

Before humor therapy or PNI were widely accepted, Norman Cousins wrote of his own experiences and became the most recognized proponent for the movement until his death in 1999. He related his personal story that he was diagnosed with a life threatening collagen disease and found conventional cures of no help. He decided to leave the hospital and checked into a hotel room where he watched endless episodes of Three Stooge movies and laughed himself to tears and recovery. He also included vitamin C in his regiment of care. Cousins, a layperson, wrote an article that was published in the New England Journal of Medicine in December 1976 which was responded to by more than three thousand doctors on the holistic health philosophy that Cousins described. Later Cousins would qualify his claims to include not just laughter, but all positive emotions as curative to the human body and spirit. He continued to write of the healing effects of laughter and the human dimension of healing in his first book, Anatomy of an Illness As Perceived by the Patient, which was an extension of the original article. Cousins was the editor for the Saturday Review, and the author of eleven books. His message was a persuasive one and his credibility already established before he began addressing the state of the medical profession in the 1970s. He said that a hospital was a terrible place to be for a truly sick person. Cousins wrote of a basic lack of sanitation, the spread of staphylococci and other pathogens, overuse of X-ray equipment, indiscriminate use of tranquilizers and painkillers, and intrusions on patients' needed sleep. Most of this he concluded was for the convenience of the staff, certainly not the patient.[7] Until his recent death, many years after the illness was supposed to kill him, Cousins remained an inspiration to people who did not respond to traditional medical routines. He discussed the bonds between emotional and physical health in the foreword to the book written by Steven Locke and Douglas Colligan, The Healer Within: The New Medicine of Mind and Body. He cited Dr. Franz Ingelfinger, former editor of the New England Journal of Medicine who estimated that 85% of human illnesses are curable by the body's own healing system.[8] We have known for a long time that a healthy lifestyle extends life and aids the body in its fight against disease, but now we know that a positive focus in life is also important to your health.

Traditional medical treatments and conventional physicians feel uneasy or even hostile toward the notion that the patient controls the outcome of his/her disease. Frequently the miracle cures are inexplicable by any traditional curative insights. The debate is a heated one between the traditionalists in medicine and those who urge a new way of looking at the human body, mind, and spirit. Many practitioners look only at the first of these -- the body-- and their vision is a mechanistic one where certain techniques are applied like surgery, addition of fluids, or prescriptions given for drugs, wherein the trinity of body, mind, and spirit are ignored.

Cousins writings were criticized by some who found his theories contrary to sound medical practices and some had used the work of Dr. Cassileth to attack Cousins' work. So Dr. Cassileth from the UCLA School of Medicine issued a statement to clarify some research which had been misinterpreted concerning the mind-body link and the interdependence between good spirits, positive emotions, purpose and determination, hope, and laughter in combating disease. Dr. Cassileth's statement made the following points:

- Emotions and health are closely related;

- Probably numerous emotional and physical factors influence health and disease;

- Positive attitudes affect the quality of life even where they cannot influence the physical outcome of the disease;

- Panic, not uncommon when cancer is diagnosed is, in itself, destructive and can interfere with effective treatment.[9]

Cousins wrote about Dr. Harold Benjamin who believed in the importance of the environmental factor in treating cancer. Benjamin established a wellness community for cancer patients where they could gather to talk and share their emotional needs. The results were that with few exceptions, the members have outlived their physician's predictions about when they would die.

The recent movie in the U.S. starring Robin Williams, Patch Adams, offered a humorous look at the issues of doctor-patient relationships, medical school protocol, and the healing effects of laughter. The movie depicts Patch dancing with bedpans on his feet and clowning around for the children in the cancer ward only to be rebuked by the Dean of the medical school. Throughout the movie, the healing effect of human connections with love, laughter, and competent medical care was portrayed with cancer patients too young to know their fate, angry, frightened adults who did, and doctors whose philosophy of treatment varied from the ridiculous to the sublime. The thesis of the movie was that laughter is healing and humans respond to loving attention, even those who are terminally ill. We do not maintain that the medical community has failed, but we do need to move beyond the body/mind dichotomy to encompass a holistic approach to healing which includes respect for people as total human beings. The movie was based upon the life of a real Patch Adams who uses humor therapy with patients.

Paul Martin discussed the historic threads of thought separating the mind and body that have ushered in the dualism in medicine in his book The Healing Mind, The Vital Links Between Brain and Behavior, Immunity and Disease.[10] Dualism has always been prominent in Western thought, but to the ancient Greek philosophers, the distinction between mind and body were not absolute. Alcmaeon, Epicurus, and Hippocrates questioned beliefs about disembodied spirits and offered explanations for the natural world in terms of observable, physical phenomena. Hippocrates born 460 B.C., whose name lives on in the medical oath, was the most prominent physician of his time. He was called the Father of Medicine. Rather than resorting to the usual explanations of the gods and evil spirits, he sought explanations based upon natural causes. Hippocratic medicine depended upon a harmonious balance of humors (blood, phlegm, yellow bile and black bile) and diseases were caused by an imbalance between these elements. Hippocrates believed that diseases were caused by natural forces that could be studied and explained. He preceded psychoneuroimmunology by over two thousand years by arguing that the mind is one of the adaptive forces that influences the body's health and response to physical disease.[11]

Galen, who was born about 130 A.D., was the foremost medical authority in the Western world and physician to the gladiators and emperor Marcus Aurelius. He established the use of the pulse as an aid to diagnosis. Like his Greek predecessors, he emphasized the rational, materialistic approach to treating disease. To Galen, "diseases were abnormal physical conditions of a physical body and not aberrations of the soul or punishments meted out by an angry deity."[12] The Greek's materialistic approach included an acknowledged existence of the psyche --the spirit, soul or mind, depending upon the translation of it. But the focus of their treatment was almost exclusively upon the physical body, the soma. But at least during this time, they acknowledged the union of the mind and body. As the clock winds forward into the Middle Ages, church dogma took us back to sin as the cause of disease. This line of thought continued until the Fifteenth and Sixteenth Century when the scientific approach to medicine was reawakening. An English physician, William Harvey, discovered how blood circulates within the body disproving many of Galen's teachings about the blood and heart.

Rene Descartes, the Seventeenth century French philosopher and mathematician was most influential in solidifying the duality of the mind and body in Western thought. Descartes used mind and soul synonymously and he argued that the mind was a nonphysical entity, implanted in the human body by God. The mind was responsible for conscious thought and this was the very essence of human existence. Cogito, ergo sum--I think; therefore, I am or I exist. According to Descartes the mind had no location and was not dependent upon the brain or any other physical, material thing. Descartes' theories gave a philosophical system that reconciled religious belief with scientific reason, thus formalizing the split between emotions and the body, or mind and body, for the next three hundred years. Martin wrote, "The Cartesian notion of a disembodied, rational mind, unencumbered by mere emotion, simply does not correspond with the true nature of the human organism. We are no more capable of coping with life solely by rational calculations than we could through emotions and feelings alone. Both are essential if we are to function in the real world."[13]

In the last decade, there has been a movement toward recognizing the role that regeneration of mind and spirit plays in one's total health. Writers have examined the prevalent attitudes toward aging and many state that the attributes that we often associate with age are not inevitable at all, but generally result from unhealthy lifestyles such as smoking, poor nutrition, and abuse of drugs or alcohol. Depak Chopra, M.D. sees life as an ongoing process of change and renewal. In his book, Ageless Body, Timeless Mind he stated:

In order to stay alive, your body must live on the wings of change. At this moment you are exhaling atoms of hydrogen, oxygen, carbon and nitrogen that just an instant before were locked up in solid matter; your stomach, liver, heart, lungs and brain are vanishing into thin air, being replaced as quickly and endlessly as they are being broken down. The skin replaces itself once a month, the stomach lining every five days, the liver every six weeks, and the skeleton every three months. To the naked eye, these organs look the same from moment to moment, but they are always in flux. By the end of this year, 98 percent of the atoms in your body will have been exchanged for new ones.[14]

Chopra noted that over time, beginning at age 30 imperceptible changes occur at about 1 percent per year. Wrinkles appear, skin tone diminishes, muscle tissues diminish, while fat increases, stamina decreases, and biochemicals cease to work at optimal levels. The results are heart disease as cholesterol rises or cellular mutations produce malignant tumors which strike one in three persons after age 65. Chopra wrote:

> Over time, these various 'age changes' as gerontologists call them, exert massive influence. They are the thousand tiny waves that bring in the tide of old age. But at any given moment, aging accounts for only 1 percent per year of the total change taking place inside your body. In other words, 99 percent of the energy and intelligence that you are composed of is untouched by the aging process. In terms of the body as process eliminating this 1 percent of dysfunction would wipe out aging. But how do we get at this 1 percent? To answer that, we must find the control switch that manipulates the body's inner intelligence.[15]

Inherent in Chopra's view are the principles that the mind and body are energy fields that change forms and that mind and body are inseparably one. People can experience the same stimulus, pain, and each will interpret it differently. For example, two patients with angina pectoris, the squeezing pain of heart disease, respond in opposite ways. One may swim, run, and feel no pain while the other almost faints with pain getting out of his armchair. Patients with 85% blockage have run marathons, he said.

These dramatic differences in individuals and the way they interpret the world tell us that we have powers to heal ourselves which we have not yet explored. Biofeedback techniques can be taught and patients can regulate blood pressure, heart rate, breathing, and pain–even the time that they die.

Our most basic bodily processes respond to our state of mind. When we read an article or story that makes us angry or afraid, our body prepares us for a fight or to take flight with adrenaline and glucose surging through our veins. Our muscles tense, breathing is more rapid, and we are energized. When we read a funny story or see a comical movie, entertainer, or event, we laugh–sometimes until we cry. And we feel better.

The ancient Greeks formalized theater which has its roots in their religious rituals. Tragedy was the highest form of theater for the Greeks believed that catharsis cleansed the soul. If the viewer could identify with the protagonist in a tragedy and be moved to feel fear or pity, then the soul was redeemed. Similarly, in comedy, the social order was imposed upon citizens or reinforced by holding up human's mistakes or character flaws such as pride, greed or stupidity for the entire society to ridicule through laughter. Laughter is redemptive for the individual mentally, physically, and socially. It reaffirms our optimism in the future. The best formula is to be able to laugh at our own mistakes instead of allowing our failures to gnaw at our hearts or psyche.

Doctors talk about patients with the cancer personality, a repressed individual who carries the burdens of life without expression or confrontation. The anger, disappointment, or grief become internalized and illness results. A 76-year old woman volunteered at her senior center every day running the coffee fund, organizing raffles and other activities which supported the center in substantial ways. She began doing these things after her 8-year-old granddaughter died from cancer. The grandmother went through a massive depression. "How could God allow someone so beautiful, so innocent, to die?" she wept. Her priest told her to get involved in giving to others and her grief would dissipate. She told this writer that only by reaching out to others did she rediscover herself and peace.

Not all of life is a laughing matter. We know that personal loss and shattered dreams wear heavily upon our soul. Reversals in health and life's fortunes come to every door eventually. What makes the difference in the final analysis is how we deal with our losses or the conclusions that we draw from them. Some believe that God is punishing them, others believe that they must be bad people and deserve these episodes, and others rant and rail at everyone close to them as the culprits who have pulled the plagues down upon them. What appears to be a special grace is possessed by those who reach into their inner core and find strength, compassion, and understanding to transcend the ravages of disease, personal loss or chaos. Some of the great artists have had tragic lives and yet found expression in the creation of beautiful music, paintings, or literature that records the essence of their lives.

On average, children laugh 400 times a day, while adults laugh only 15 times a day.[16] Somewhere between childhood and adulthood, we lose about 385 laughs a day. We may ask ourselves where the laughter has gone. Children still delight in encountering others, exploring new places, trying new things, and exercising their imagination. Adults grow weary of all the restrictions that a politically correct environment requires and we grow tired from all the pressures of everyday life. Like the river rocks which have been rounded from all the water washing over them and wearing them into similar shapes, adults have been worn down by the storms that assault us through life. Yet some retain the ability to see humor in the trials and tribulations that absolutely kneel others. For some reason they generally find something humorous in situations where there is supposed to be decorum and solemnity like church services, a funeral, or a wedding. We all have stories that we enjoy retelling where an embarrassing incident occurred and someone had the capacity to make the most of it. For example, the minister who was standing at grave side and slipped into the hole. He jumped out, spread his arms before the amazed crowd and declared, "I have risen!" A similar incident occurred at a wedding where a woman signing the guest registry near a candle caught her chiffon laced hat on fire. When a male companion began beating her over the head with a newspaper to extinguish the fire, she almost decked him. Had they not been so regally dressed, the scene would not have been so funny. So we laugh when someone is being ridiculous, or to relieve nervous tension, and when we see something unexpected or incongruous.

According to Lee Berk, assistant research professor, and Stanley Tan,

Endocrinologist and their colleagues, at California's Loma Linda University Medical Center, there are two types of stress: good stress and bad stress. Laughter is a good form of stress which reverses the bad stressors that suppress your immune system. Here is what they found after studying two groups of average adults with one group having a solid hour of induced merriment from videos of comedians, while the other group did not. The doctors took blood samples at 10 minute intervals before and during and after the exposure to funny videos. This is quoted directly from Crystal and Flanagan.

> They found that humor and exercise trigger similar physiological processes. Like conditioned athletes, the laughter group showed increases in the good hormones - such as endorphins and neurotransmitters – and decreased levels of the stress hormones – cortisol and adrenaline. Laughter is one of the body's safety valves, a counter balance to tension. When we release that tension, the elevated levels of the body's stress hormones drop back to normal, thereby allowing our immune systems to work more effectively. Cells which produce anti-bodies increase in number, T-cells which combat viruses are activated and ready for battle. Our natural killer cells increase in number and activity. All this occurs as a direct result of laughter.[17]

Even though many critics say these studies have too few subjects, or that it is hard to separate the elements that are operating at that time to determine cause and effect, The medical community is taking this type of research seriously. Psychiatrist Robert Holden, who is a recognized stress consultant, runs laughter clinics for England's National Health Service where over 5,000 health care professionals have attended training events. Holden was quoted as saying "Your day goes the way the corners of your mouth turn,"[18] He said since it is possible for all 400 muscles in your body to move when you laugh, laughter has been labeled as internal aerobics. If you could sustain a belly laugh for an hour, you could burn off 500 calories. When we laugh, we produce endorphins ('of morphine') which are the body's natural relaxants that stimulate feelings of well being, joy and a high. Holden said we do not stop laughing because we become old; we become old because we stop laughing.[19] Many hospitals now have a comedy channel on television for all of their patients to view.

Laughter is a form of internal jogging. It should be exercised regularly for maximum effect. There is irrefutable evidence to support the benefits of laughter to the mind and body of every individual as well as society in general. According to William F. Fry, M.D., Professor of Psychiatry at Stanford University Medical School, 20 seconds of robust laughter works the heart like 3 minutes of hard rowing and 100 laughs a day gives you the physical benefits of riding a stationary bike for 15 minutes.[20]

A writer once noted that there are three responses to life– Aha!, Ah!, and Ha Ha! -- Aha! Or Eureka, means enlightenment has occurred. Perhaps a problem has been solved or a solution found for an issue that has troubled us for some time. Suddenly like the proverbial light bulb clicking on, we seem to fall upon a worthy idea. The Ah! response represents the wonder of a child engrossed in something absorbing like a sunbeam or a butterfly. We lose our capacity to appreciate our interpersonal and physical environment sometimes. Watch two and three-year olds as they explore their garden path and you will find a whole new world beneath your feet. The final response is Ha-Ha!, or laughter. The merits of a chuckle or convulsive laughter are apparent to anyone who remembers how it feels. Laughter is good medicine and the cathartic effect of it has been known since the early Greeks.

Like the thunder that reverberates through the canyons and the lightening that accompanies it, our laughter sends a surge of energy not unlike the electromagnetic fields in nature. It is powerful and produces flashes of brilliance that light up dark recesses of our soul as well as the lives of others.

We need to become reacquainted with what Steven Locke, and Douglas Colligan call "the healer within."[21] Their premise is that the immune system, our best line of defense, does not exist in a vacuum driven by the lymphatic system. The immune system is linked to the brain, our organ of thought, a relationship which is demonstrated through the evolving branch of research discussed earlier as psychoneuroimmunology. The whole concept returns us to a holistic view of humans and medicine. We are not pieces or organs to be scrutinized microscopically and treated incrementally. We are a unified whole who thinks, feels, and changes dynamically as we interact with our environment and others while we negotiate the shoals of sickness and unhappiness to find solace and refuge in troubled times. On this high ground, laughter can be heard frequently and a feeling of being part of something much bigger permeates our consciousness.

Endnotes

1. Dacher, E. S. (1991a). <u>PNI the new mind body healing program</u>. New York: Paragon House.

2. Dacher, E. S. (1991b). <u>PNI the new mind body healing program</u>. (p. 21.) New York: Paragon House.

3. Dacher, E. S. (1991c). <u>PNI the new mind body healing program</u>. (p. 15.) New York: Paragon House.

4. Dacher, E. S. (1991d). <u>PNI The New Mind Body Healing Program</u>. New York: Paragon House.

5. Dacher, E. S. (1991e). <u>PNI the new mind body healing program</u>. (p. 17.) New York: Paragon House.

6. Dacher, E. S. (1991f). <u>PNI the new mind body healing program</u>. New York: Paragon House.

7. Cousins, N. (1979). <u>Anatomy of an illness as perceived by the patient</u>. New York: W. W. Norton & Company

8. Cousins, N. (1986a). Foreword. In Locke, S., & Colligan, D. <u>The healer within:The new medicine of mind and body</u>.(p. ix). New York: E. P. Dutton.

9. Cousins, N. (1986a). Foreword. In Locke, S., & Colligan, D. <u>The healer within:The new medicine of mind and body</u>.(p. ix). New York: E. P. Dutton.

10. Martin, P. (1998a). <u>The healing mind the vital links between brain and Behavior Immunity and Disease</u>. New York: St Martin's Press.

11. Martin, P. (1998b). <u>The healing mind the vital links between brain and behavior immunity and disease</u>. (P. 269). New York: St. Martin's Press.

12. Martin, P. (1998b). <u>The healing mind the vital links between brain and behavior immunity and disease</u>. (P. 270). New York: St. Martin's Press.

13. Martin, P. (1998b). <u>The healing mind the vital links between brain and behavior immunity and disease</u>. (P. 273). New York: St. Martin's Press.

14. Chopra, D. (1993a). <u>Ageless body timeless mind the quantum alternative to growing old.</u> (P. 9). New York: Harmony Books

130

15. Chopra, D. (1993a). <u>Ageless body timeless mind the quantum alternative to growing old.</u> (P. 10). New York: Harmony Books

16. Crystal, G., & Flanagan, P. (1995a). <u>Laughter-Still the best medicine.</u> (p 1-2). <u>Available: http://www.heylady.com/rbc/laughter.htm.</u>

17. Crystal, G., & Flanagan, P. (1995b). <u>Laughter-Still the best medicine.</u> (p 1-2). <u>Available: http://www.heylady.com/rbc/laughter.htm.</u>

18. Holden, R. (1998a, April). A dose of laughter medicine. <u>Stress News, 10, 2.</u> (On line) <u>http://www.15ma.org.uk/Laughter.htm.</u>

19. Holden, R. (1998b, April). A dose of laughter medicine. <u>Stress News, 10, 2.</u> (On line) <u>http://www.15ma.org.uk/Laughter.htm.</u>

20. Foltz-Gray, D. (1998, November December). Comic relief. <u>Arthritis Today. 12 6.</u> p. 26-30.

21. Locke, S., and Colligan, D.(1986c). <u>The healer within the new medicine of mind and body.</u> New York: E. P. Dutton.

Bibliography

Accidents and the elderly. National Institute on Aging Age Page. U.S.
    Department of Health and Human Services.
    http://www.mfaaa.org/center/agepage/accident_eld.html.

Ader, R., Felten, D. A., & Cohen, N. (Eds.) (1991). Psychoneuroimmunology. (2nd
    ed.), San Diego: Academic Press.

Aging, drugs and alcohol. (1995). Encyclopedia of drugs and alcohol. J. H. Jaffe,
    (Ed.), (Vol 1. pp. 51-58). New York: Macmillan Library Reference USA.

Alston, S., & Silverthorne-McIntosh, S. (1991). Use it or lose it. Public Health
    Reports, 106, 212-213.

American Heart Association (1999, June 22,)New unified dietary guidelines
    offer nutritional protection against wide range of killer diseases. Available
    http:www.sciencedaily.com/releases/1999/06/990622061026.htm

Atkins, R. C., & Gare, F. (1997). Dr. Atkins New Diet Cookbook. New York:
    M. Evans and Company, Inc.

Bandura, A. L. (1989). Human agency in social cognitive theory. American
    Psychologist 44, 1175-1184.

Bendall, M. J., Basser, E. J., & Pearson, M. B. (1989). Factors affecting walking
    speed of elderly people. Age and Ageing 18, 327-332.

Black, J., & Bryant, J. (1995). Introduction to communication. (4th ed.), Dubuque,
    IA: Brown & Benchmark Publishers.

Burdman, G. M. (1986). Healthful aging. Englewood Cliffs, NJ: Prentice Hall.

Burns, J., Sneddon, I., Lovell, M., McLean, A., & Martin, B. J. (1992). Elderly
    patients and their medications: A post discharge follow-up study. Age and
    Ageing 21, 178-181.

132

Carpenter, D. (1993). A review and new look at ethical suicide in advanced age. The Gerontologist, 33, 359-365.

Carruthers, S. G. (1983). Clinical pharmacology of aging. In R. D. T. Cape, R. M. Coe, & I Rossman (Eds.) In Fundamentals of geriatric medicine, (pp.187-196). New York: Raven Press.

Chopra, D. (1993). Ageless body timeless mind: The quantum alternative to growing old. New York: Harmony Books.

Cohen-Sachs, B. (1993, January). Coping with the stress of aging creatively. Stress Medicine, 9, 45-49.

Cousins, N. (1979). Anatomy of an illness as perceived by the patient. New York: W. W. Norton & Company.

Cousins, N. (1983). The healing heart:Antidotes to panic and helplessness. New York: W. W. Norton & Company.

Cox, H. G. (1993). Later life: The realities of aging, (3rd ed.). Englewood Cliffs, NJ: Simon and Schuster.

Crandall, R. C. (1991). Gerontology: A behavioral science approach. New York: McGraw-Hill.

Crystal, G., & Flanagan, P. (1995). Laughter - Still the best medicine. Available: http://www.heylady.com/rbc/laughter.htm.

Dacher, E., & Elliott, S. (1989). Peace, love & healing. New York: Harper & Row.

Davis, L., & Knutson, K. D. (1991). Warning signals for malnutrition in the elderly. Journal of the American Dietetic Association, 91, 1413-1417.

DiGiovanna, A. G. (1994). Human Aging: Biological perspectives. New York: McGraw-Hill.

Eades, M. R., & Eades, M. D. (1996) Protein power. New York: Bantam Books.

Edlin,, G., & Golanty, E. (1988). Health & wellness: A holistic approach. (3rd ed.). Boston: Jones and Bartlett.

Elderly rate hazards at home. (1990, August). USA Today Newsview, 119, 2543. 12-13.

Folkenberg, J. (1990). Testing drugs in older people. FDA Consumer, 24, 24-27.

Friedan, B. (1994, March 20). How to live longer, better, wiser. Parade Magazine, 4-6.

Generations special issue on alcohol and drug abuse: Abuse and misuse. (1998, Summer). American Society on Aging, 64-65.

Gibran, K. (1996). The Prophet. New York: Alfred A. Knopf Publisher (original work published 1923)

Goldberg, J., Beeson, L. L., Darbous, P., & Getto, M. (1990). Assistive technology in personal care service. Harrisburg, PA: PA Department of Aging.

Greeley, A. (1990, October). Nutrition and the elderly. FDA Consumer. 25-28.

Greiger, L. AHA dietary guidelines for a healthy heart. Heart Information Network. Copyright 1996-2000 Center for Cardiovascular Education, Inc., New Providence, NJ. USA http://www.heartinfo.org/nutrition/dietguide1101000.htm.

Hall, E. T. (1983). The dance of life: The other dimension of time. New York: Anchor Press/Doubleday.

134

Harris, D. R. (Ed). (1996). <u>Diet and nutrition sourcebook. Vol 15.</u> Bellenir, K.
(Series Ed.) Health Reference Series. Penobscot Building: Detroit: MI:
Omnigraphics, Inc., Frederick G. Ruffner, Jr., Publisher.

Henry, R. R., & Edleman S. V. (1992). Advances in treatment of type II diabetes
mellitus in the elderly. <u>Geriatrics. 47.</u> 24-30.

Humphrey, D. (2000, November 12). Prisoner of conscience Dr. Jack Kevorkian,
prisoner #284797 Martyr to the cause of the right to choose to die.
http::// finalexit.org.dr.K.html. E-mail: <u>efto@efn.org.</u>

Improving the odds. (1991). <u>Harvard Health Letter. 16. 4.</u>

<u>Insel. P. M.. & Roth</u>, W. T. (1988). <u>Core concepts in health</u>. Palo Alto, CA:
Mayfield Publishing Co.

Inside "Dr. Koop's Community": Q&A with C. Everett Koop. (1998, July 22)
<u>Business Week Online.</u> Copyright 1998. The McGraw-Hill Companies, Inc.
http://www.businessweek.com/bwdaily/dnflash/july1998/nf80722e.htm

Jampolsky, G., & Cirincione, D. V. (1993). <u>Change your mind change your life.</u>
Nw York: Bantam Books.

Kahl, A., Blandford, D. H., Krueger, K., Zwick, D. I. (1992, January/February).
Geriatric education centers address medication issues affecting older
adults. <u>Public Health Reports. 107.</u> 37-47.

Keller, D. New American Heart Association dietary guidelines.
<u>Http://www.wellnessweb.com/HEART/ahadiet.htm.</u> E-mail
WellnessWeb.

Key, S.W., (Ed.) & Marble, M. Unified dietary guidelines offer nutritional
protection against fatal diseases. (1999, July 12 & 19). <u>Cancer Weekly
Plus. CWHenderson Publisher.</u> 15.

Krause, N. (1991). Stressful events and life satisfaction among elderly men and
women. <u>Journal of Gerontology: Social Sciences 46.</u> 84-92.

Kuhn, M., Long, C., & Quinn, L. (1991). No stone unturned: The life and times of Maggie Kuhn. New York: Ballantine Books.

Lefcourt, H.M., & Martin, R. A. (1986). Humor and life stress. New York: Springer-Verlag.

Leonard, G. B. (1968). Education and ecstasy. New York: Delacorte Press.

Lindley, C. M., Tully, M. P., Paramsothy, V., & Tallis, R. C. (1992). Inappropriate medication is a major cause of adverse drug reactions in elderly patients. Age and Ageing, 21, 294-300.

Locke, S., & Colligan, D. (1986). The healer within. New York: E. P. Dutton.

Lowery, S.A., & DeFleur, M. L. (1995). Milestones in Mass Communication Research. (3rd ed.). Needham Heights, MA: Pearson Education.

Lucas, S.E. (1995). The art of public speaking. (5th ed.). New York: Random House.

Martin, P. (1998). The healing mind the vital links between brain and Behavior Immunity and Disease. New York: St Martin's Press.

Mazer, C. M. University of Pennsylvania. Bernard Shaw: a brief biography. http://www.english.upenn.edu/~cmazer/mis1.html.

Michigan v. Dr. Jack Kevorkian. Court Library. http://www.courttv.com/casefiles/verdicts/kevorkian.html

Nappi, G., Genazzani, A. R., Martigmani, E., & Petraglia, F. (1990). Stress and the aging brain: Integrative mechanisms. New York: Raven Press.

National Institute on Aging. Accidents and the elderly.(1991). Age Page a. U. S. Department of Health and Human Services, NIA Information Center P. O. Box - Gaithersburg, MD 20898-8057. Available: http://www.mfaa.org/center/agepage/accident_eld.html

136

National Institute on Drug Abuse. (1988). Biological vulnerability to drug abuse (Research Monograph, 89. Washington, DC: U. S. Printing Office.

New unified dietary guidelines offer nutritional protection against wide range of killer diseases. (1999, June 22). American Heart Association. Http://www.americanheart.org. http://www.sciencedaily.com/releases/1999/06/990622061026.htm

Neugarten, B., Havighurst, R., & Tobin, S. (1968). Personality and patterns of aging. In B. Neugarten (Ed.), Middle age and aging (pp.173-78). Chicago: University of Chicago Press.

Newbern, V. B. (1991) Is it really Alzheimers? American Journal of Nursing, 91, 50-56.

Nutrition of the elderly. (1992 January/February). Nutrition Today, 27, 33-34.

O'Neill, C. J. A., Dobbs, R. J., Dobbs, S. M., & Nicholson, P. W. (1991). Measurements of compliance with medication: The sine qua non of clinical trials in old age? Age and Ageing, 20, 77-79.

Parker, S. L. (1992). National survey of nutritional risk among the elderly. Journal of Nutrition Education, 24, 238.

Payne, W. A., Hahn, D. B., & Pinger, R. R. (1991). Drugs: Issues for today. Baltimore: Mosby Year Book.

Persson, D. (1993). The elderly driver: Deciding when to stop. The Gerontologist, 33, 88-91.

Porterfield, J. D., & St. Pierre, R. (1992). Wellness: Healthful aging. Guilford, CT: Dushkin.

Ray, O., & Ksir, C. (1993). Drugs, society, & human behavior. (7th ed.), St. Louis, MO: Mosby Year Book.

Rosenfield, I. (1985). Modern prevention: The new medicine. New York: Simon & Schuster.

Rubin, A. (2000, October 10). Proper nutrition and the elderly. e-mail
RehabStrat@aol.com orrubin@brainlink.com.
http://www.therubins.com/aging/diet/htm

Ruth, J., & P. (1996). Personality and aging: Coping and management of the self
in later life. In J. E. Birren and Schaie (Eds.), Handbook of the psychology
of aging (pp.308-322). New York: Van Nostrand Reinhold.

Rybash, J., Roodin, P., & Santrock, J. (1991). Adult development and aging (2nd
ed.), IO: Wm C. Brown.

Safety program reduces risk of home accidents. (1989). Aging, 359, 35-36.

Siegel, B. S. (1986). Love medicine & miracles: Lessons learned about self-
healing from a surgeon's experience with exceptional patients. New York:
Harper and Row.

Siegel, B. S. (1989). Peace, love & healing: Bodymind communication and the
path to self-healing: An exploration. New York: Harper & Row.

Simpson, J. B. (1988). Simpson's contemporary quotations. Boston: Houghton
Mifflin Co.

Steward, H. L., Morrison, C. B., Andrews, S. S., & Balart, L. A. (1995). Sugar
busters! Cut sugar to trim fat. New York: Ballantine Books.

Strength training helps frail elderly. (1994). Health and Human Development
Home Page Penn State Home Page. Available:
http://www.hhdev.psu.edu/research/Strength.htm

Timiras, P. S. (1994a). Aging of the adrenal and pituitary. In P. S. Timiras (Ed.),
Physiological basis of aging and geriatrics (2ND ed.). pp. 133-146.
Boca Raton, FL: CRC Press.

Timiras, P. S. (1994b). Aging of the nervous system: Functional Changes. In P.
S. Timiras (Ed.), Physiological basis of aging and geriatrics (2nd ed.).
pp.103-114. Boca Raton, FL: CRC Press.

138

Tyson, P. (1999, May). Laughter is the best medicine. (Making children laugh) Sesame Street Magazine. http://www.findarticles.com/m0GDK/1999_May/54504257/p1/article.jhtm l.

USDAUnited States Department of Agriculture News Release, (2000, May 27). USDAm HHS release updated dietary guidelines for Americans. United States Department of Health and Human Services.Government Printing Office or the Consumer Information Center. Stock number 001-000-046681-1. http://www.health.gov/dietatyguidelines/dga2000/pressrelease.htm

U. S. Department of Census. (1995). Statistical Abstract of the United States (115 ed., p. 16). Washington, DC .

U. S. Food and Drug Administration. (1999). Eating well as we age. (Publication No. 99-2311). Rockville, MD: Author.

Van Loon, G. R., Kvetnansky, R., McCarty, R., & Axwelrod, J. (1989). Stress, neurochemical and humoral mechanisms, ISMS (Vol. 1). New York: Gordon and Breach Science.

Walker, D., & Beuchene, R. E. (1991). The relationship of loneliness, social isolation, and physical health to dietary adequacy of independently living elderly. Journal of the American Dietetic Association, 91, 300-304.

Wolfe, S., Hope, R, & Public Citizen Health Research Group. (1993). Worst pills best pills: The older adult's guide to avoiding drug-induced death or illness. Washington, DC: Public Citizen's Health Research Group.

Work, J. A. (1991). Strength training: A bridge to independence for the elderly. Physician & Sports Medicine, 17 (11), 134-140.

World Almanac and Book of Facts 1996. (1995). Mahwah, NJ: Funk and Wagnalls Corporation.

Young, V. R. (1990). Amino acids and proteins in relation to the nutrition of elderly people. Age and Ageing, 19, 10-24.

Name Index

Word Index

142

STUDIES IN HEALTH AND HUMAN SERVICES